Y0-ACH-677

PSYCHIATRIC SERVICES IN THE COMMUNITY: DEVELOPMENTS AND INNOVATIONS

Psychiatric Services in the Community

Developments and Innovations

Edited by
JOHN REED and GILLIAN LOMAS

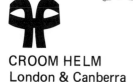

CROOM HELM
London & Canberra

© 1984 John Reed and Gillian Lomas
Croom Helm Ltd, Provident House, Burrell Row,
Beckenham, Kent BR3 1AT
Croom Helm Australia Pty Ltd, 28 Kembla St.,
Fyshwick, ACT 2609, Australia

British Library Cataloguing in Publication Data

Psychiatric service in the community
    1. Community mental health services. —
    Great Britain
    I. Reed, John   II. Lomas, Gillian
    362.2'0941   RA790.7.G7

    ISBN 0-7099-2264-7

Printed and bound in Great Britain by
Biddles Ltd, Guildford and King's Lynn

CONTENTS

Foreword   8
      Ian Kelsey-Fry

Contributors   9

Introduction   13
      John Reed and Gillian Lomas

PART ONE   19
THE IDEAS AND POLICIES BEHIND THE DEVELOPMENT
OF COMPREHENSIVE LOCAL SERVICES

 1 Developments in Community Psychiatry: 21
    A Central View
         Lord Trefgarne
    Discussion and Comments by R H Cawley

 2 Information for Psychiatric Services   31
         Neil Zammett and Jill Sternfeld

 3 Training in Community Psychiatry   39
         Sam Baxter

 4 Ethical Issues in Community-based   44
    Psychiatry
         Ian E Thompson

 5 Straightening the Bend: Sociological   55
    Contributions towards the Development
    of Community Mental Health Care
         Geoffrey Baruch

 6 The Stigma of Psychiatric Disorder: 67
    A Sociological Perspective and Research
    Report
         Agnes Miles

PART TWO   75
PLANNING THE IDEAL SERVICE: CLINICAL AND
NON-CLINICAL ELEMENTS

 7 The Elements of an Ideal Service: 77
    The Clinical View
        John Reed
    Discussion and Comments by Bernard Heine

 8 A House for all Reasons: 91
    The Role of Housing in Community Care
        Adrian Lovett
    Discussion and Comments by Ian Diamant

 9 Planning an Ideal Service for Newham: 105
    The Problems
        Deirdre Cunningham

10 Fitting the Jigsaw Together   110
        K A M Grant

11 The Nursing Element in an Ideal Service   114
        Paul G Beard

12 Planning a Psychiatric Intensive Care Unit   121
        Ruth Seifert

13 The Gentle Touch: Principles for Progress   128
        Gillian Lomas

PART THREE   137
THE ELEMENTS PUT INTO PRACTICE

14 Services in the Net   139
        Donald H Dick
    Discussion and Comments by Edith Morgan

15 Rehabilitation and Community Care: 153
    Working Together
        Mark A J O'Callaghan

16 A Worm's Eye View: 164
    Experiences as an Administrator
        Frank Osborn

17 Brindle House: A Community   171
    Mental Health Service in Practice
        Roger Hargreaves

18 Psychiatric Illness in General Practice   178
        Anthony W Clare

19 Day Hospital for Dementia: 191
        Safety Net for a High-wire Act?
        Susan Hodgson

PART FOUR   197
CONSOLIDATION: LOOKING TO THE FUTURE

20 The Myth of Sisyphus: Turning   199
        Mountains into Molehills
        Chris Heginbotham

21 Where are we now? Summary and Conclusions   211
        Douglas Bennett

BIBLIOGRAPHY   215
        compiled by Geoffrey Baruch

INDEX   247

FOREWORD

I was very pleased when Dr Reed asked me to chair a
session at the conference organised by the Community
Psychiatry Research Unit on the development of
comprehensive district services for the mentally
ill. It is equally a pleasure to write a foreword to
this book based on the proceedings of that
conference.

When the conference was planned the organisers
cannot have known that it would open on such an
auspicious day for St Bartholomew's Hospital Medical
College. As it turned out, there were two
significant events on that day. While Lord
Trefgarne, then Parliamentary Under Secretary at the
Department of Health and Social Security, was
delivering the opening paper at the conference on
psychiatric services, Mr Geoffrey Finsburg, another
Minister, was opening a new clinical research
centre. It seemed particularly striking that the
wide range of interests of the Medical College was
so elegantly illustrated on the same day.

Ten years ago, of course, one event would have
been regarded as much more important than the other;
there is little doubt as to which that would have
been. Now the situation is quite different. The
Medical College recognises the great benefits of
having a wider involvement the community around it,
and understands the important role an academic
institution can play. It is essential that our
students and doctors hear about the sort of work
discussed in this book and play an active part in
it. I am very glad that the Medical College has been
able to be a focus for this exciting, pioneering
work.

Dr Ian Kelsey-Fry
Dean, The Medical College,
St Bartholomew's Hospital, London, EC 1.

CONTRIBUTORS

Geoffrey BARUCH PhD
Research worker, Community Psychiatry Research Unit, Hackney Hospital.

Dr Sam BAXTER
Consultant Psychiatrist, Hammersmith & Fulham DHA and Charing Cross Hospital.

Paul G BEARD
Director of Nursing Services (Mental Health), Bloomsbury District Health Authority.

Dr Douglas BENNETT
Consultant Psychiatrist, Bethlem Royal and Maudsley Hospitals.

Professor R H CAWLEY
Joint Professor of Psychological Medicine, King's College Hospital Medical School and Institute of Psychiatry.

Professor Anthony W CLARE
Head, Department of Psychological Medicine, St Bartholomew's Hospital Medical College.

Dr Deirdre CUNNINGHAM
Senior Registrar in Community Medicine, St Thomas' Hospital Medical School, London.

Ian DIAMANT
Special Projects Officer, London and Quadrant Housing Trust.

Dr D H DICK
Consultant Psychiatrist, Wessex Regional Health Authority (West Dorset), and formerly Director, NHS Health Advisory Service.

Dr K A M GRANT
District Medical Officer, City and Hackney District Health Authority.

Roger HARGREAVES
Senior Caseworker (Mental Health), Tameside Metropolitan Borough Council. Member of Mental Health Act Commission.

Chris HEGINBOTHAM
Director, MIND (National Association for Mental Health).

Dr Bernard HEINE
Consultant Psychiatrist, Runwell Hospital, Southend District Health Authority, and chairman, North East Thames Regional Health Authority Psychiatric Advisory Committee.

Dr Susan HODGSON
Consultant Psychogeriatrician, Withington Hospital, South Manchester District Health Authority.

Gillian LOMAS
Co-Director, Community Psychiatry Research Unit, Hackney Hospital.

Adrian LOVETT
District Comprehensive Housing Officer, London Borough of Hackney.

Agnes MILES PhD
Senior Lecturer in Medical Sociology, Department of Sociology and Social Administration, University of Southampton.

Edith MORGAN
Director, Good Practices in Mental Health Project (International Hospital Federation), Member of Mental Health Act Commission, President Elect, World Federation for Mental Health.

Mark O'CALLAGHAN
Senior Clinical Psychologist, Hollymoor Hospital and Middlewood House, Solihull Health District.

Frank OSBORN
District General Administrator, Haringey District Health Authority.

Dr John REED
Consultant Psychiatrist, St Bartholomew's and
Hackney Hospitals, Co-Director, Community Psychiatry
Research Unit.

Dr Ruth SEIFERT
Consultant Psychiatrist, St Bartholomew's and
Hackney Hospitals.

Jill STERNFELD
District Information Officer, City and Hackney
District Health Authority.

Ian E THOMPSON PhD
Senior Educationalist, Scottish Health Education
Group, Edinburgh.

Lord TREFGARNE
Parliamentary Under Secretary of State at the
Ministry of Defence, and formerly Parliamentary
Under Secretary of State at the Department of Health
and Social Security.

Neil ZAMMETT
Senior Operational Research Scientist, North West
Thames Regional Health Authority.

INTRODUCTION

John Reed and Gillian Lomas

In November 1982, the staff of the Community
Psychiatry Research Unit arranged a conference,
entitled 'Cinderella No More', to discuss the
development of comprehensive district psychiatric
services. The papers delivered at this conference
have been revised and edited so that together they
form a substantive report on the ideas, planning and
practice of community-oriented services for the
mentally ill in England. The conference was chaired
by Dr Douglas Bennett, who has provided the final
chapter for this book, and by Dr Ian Kelsey-Fry, who
has written the foreword. The Department of Health
and Social Security recognised the importance and
timeliness of the conference by suggesting that Lord
Trefgarne, then Parliamentary Under Secretary,
deliver the opening paper.

The Community Psychiatry Research Unit was
formed in 1979 to provide a focus for a co-ordinated
programme of research and action projects to improve
hospital and community services for people with
psychiatric illnesses. There are now two groups of
staff: a research and development team which also
co-ordinates housing projects and is responsible for
negotiating policy developments; and the Support
Network which offers direct support to clients. CPRU
is a unit of St Bartholomew's Hospital Medical
College and has been funded mainly with generous
grants from the Gatsby Trust. From April 1983 the
District Health Authority assumed some financial
responsibility for the unit with the intention of
incorporating it into mainline funding by 1986.

One advantage for us, as editors of a book such
as this, was to be able to prepare the introduction
after an adequate period in which to digest the
material. In this instance, the interval, although
only eight months, has been sufficient also for us

to realise that there have been many developments in
the move towards replacing outdated, poorly situated
mental illness hospitals with services located
within the community they aim to serve. The impetus
for much change has come concurrently from many
sources, the Royal College of Psychiatrists, the
Royal College of Nursing, the Department of Health
and Social Security, and COHSE, to cite but a few.
The atmosphere of change, coinciding with a crucial
period in the planning cycles of regional health
authorities, has meant that a great deal has
happened. Many districts are now able to move ahead
very actively with community-oriented services. Our
own activities, in the City and Hackney Health
District, the main example throughout the conference, have progressed in a variety of ways. For
instance, use is being made of the 'Care in the
Community' provisions (DHSS 1981, 1983b) for
improving the service for elderly mentally ill
people, and we are at present setting up a
computerised psychiatric service register, with the
help of a grant from the King Edward's Hospital
Fund.
    Documents supporting the general trend towards
locally-based services have appeared from varied
sources. DHSS itself has issued a new and important
- albeit slim - Mental Illness Policy Paper (DHSS
1983a), on which we have commented in the light of
our Hackney experience (Reed 1983). MIND, the
National Association for Mental Health, has produced
its own booklet on comprehensive local mental health
services (MIND 1983). The Department of the
Environment has published its commissioned study on
housing for mentally ill and mentally handicapped
people (Richie et al. 1983), and, in so doing, has
helped to reinforce the emphasis that we and others
place on closer involvement of statutory housing
bodies in this field. Dr Donald Dick, one of the
main conference speakers, has refined his ideas of
the elements of an ideal service (Dick 1983). The
run-down of more of the outdated large mental
illness hospitals is incorporated into the strategic
plans of several regional health authorities.
    In view of all this, this report of the
conference, 'Cinderella No More', has much to offer.
The chapters, which cover an exceedingly wide range
of topics, are directly relevant to the current
planning and delivery of comprehensive services for
mental illness.
    The aim of the conference was to bring
information about both theory and practice of

district-based psychiatric services to a wide
audience by gathering a large group of professionals
who would participate in constructive discussion,
guided by speakers actively involved in the subject.
Participants included staff from the DHSS, local
authority social services and housing departments,
from housing associations and voluntary agencies, in
addition to doctors, nurses, paramedical staff,
health service administrators and planners from
regional and district health authorities and
research workers. This book is likewise addressed to
people from many fields of interest. We hope also,
by presenting reports of projects and schemes which
are in many ways successful in caring for those with
mental illness and disability, to dispel the persistent 'Cinderella' image and persuade planners and
practitioners that community-oriented services can
both be achieved, and once working, benefit us all.
Our success on both counts can, perhaps, be judged
by reading the comments made by Dr Douglas Bennett,
in the final chapter.
    The titles and summaries at the start of each
section are sufficient introduction for a reader to
assess his likely interest. The conference itself
was organised to follow a logical sequence: firstly,
papers covering aspects of the theories, ideas and
policies upon which community-based psychiatric
services are founded; secondly, issues germane to
planning, maintaining and improving such a service;
thirdly, reports of practical methods of delivering
psychiatric care and support; and finally a look to
the future. Each conference session began with a
major paper (or, in one case, two), with an invited
discussant, covering many aspects of the main theme
of the session. These main papers were followed by a
number of seminars during which speakers led
discussion in more depth, on topics or issues which
had been raised within the main paper. The book
follows the same sequence: each of the main papers,
with comments and discussion, is followed by chapters written from the tapes made during the seminar
sessions. The final, short, chapter was compiled
from the notes which the chairman accumulated
throughout the conference.
    There are several points which pervade many
chapters and which are important enough to warrant
further emphasis here. The issues of co-ordination
and collaboration are raised in many of the
chapters, and are certainly of paramount importance
to the success of a service. There must, of course,
be some formal mechanisms - committees, usually -

for co-ordinating the planning processes, especially
of the health service and the local authorities, the
biggest spenders. Likewise there must be a formal
structure for managing the service. But it is not
enough simply to have the requisite machinery for
collaboration, when so much, in practice, depends on
personal contact between members of staff, at many
levels. We should make a conscious effort to
remember that, although interdependent, the clinical
(health service) and non-clinical (largely local
authority and voluntary organisations) elements of a
comprehensive service will generally involve very
different styles of management and be supplied by
people who would not normally meet through their
routine work. Informal contacts may well have a
substantial though intangible effect on the smooth
running of a service.

This idea bears on another point which crops up
from time to time: that of attitudes. Who listens to
whom? Who influences the development of a service?
It has been suggested that psychiatrists feel that a
scheme must be endorsed by a colleague before it is
acceptable; that members of voluntary organisations
oppose hospital services because they are controlled
by doctors; that administrators reject anything that
does not have the DHSS seal of approval. All these
are extreme statements, but there is a grain of
truth in them, indicating a situation worthy of
careful scrutiny. Again, personal contact is vital:
no-one is likely to trust a person they have never
met or spoken to.

Finally, the thorny question of finance. All
contributors were encouraged to include some discussion of the financial aspects of whatever topic
they were covering. The paucity of the discussion
and references is indicative of how ill-understood
are the various funding methods, but at least there
seems to be a consensus that money will not
substitute for careful thought. From our own
experience we suggest that effort be put into
ensuring, first of all, that funds are available to
pay for someone whose main responsibility is to be a
local advocate of district-based psychiatric
services, who can act as a focus for planning and
can, directly or indirectly, ensure that money is
found, from the wide range of available sources, to
carry out the plans. Writing research proposals,
papers for housing development committees, ap-
plications for project grants, all take skill and a
good deal of time, and should not be relegated to
the 'spare' time of an administrator, medical

officer or consultant psychiatrist.

We must, as editors, record our thanks to the speakers at our conference, who, once they had recovered from the horror of reading the transcript of their actual words, have, almost without exception, risen handsomely to the task of producing readable and intelligent chapters for publication. Only one of the conference speakers, Barbara Stocking, has been unable to contribute to the book, because of the other publishing commitments for her research. That our contributors have respected our deadlines has also made our task a pleasant one. We decided not to incorporate verbatim discussion from the seminar sessions, but rather to include important points into the text where they seemed most relevant. There is, inevitably, some overlap of subject matter; also inevitably, some contradictions in interpretation of ideas and information. We have tried to edit with a light touch, retaining the character and style of each author and refraining from moderating or amending individual views. It follows that readers who wish to take issue with any particular point should do so with the author concerned.

CPRU staff: Pam Pemberton, Alison Gomm, Jackie Herring, Dr Margaret Rich, Geoffrey Baruch and, latterly, Christine Bassam, have made inestimable contributions in many ways, in arranging the conference, and also to the many aspects of the production of this book. Joanna Reid has been our painstaking sub-editor, and has read and corrected several drafts of the text.

We would also like to record our thanks to E R Squibb and Sons for the generous donation which enabled us to prepare the bibliography for the conference which is also included in this book.

Finally, we wish to express our gratitude to Andrew Dunlop of the District Computing Unit, St Bartholomew's Hospital, whose patience and ingenuity has enabled us to make this book look elegant.

REFERENCES

DHSS (1981). Care in the Community. A Consultative Document on Moving Resources for Care in England, Circular HC(81)9/LAC(81)5.

DHSS (1983a). Mental Illness: Policies for Prevention, Treatment, Rehabilitation and Care, Mental Illness Policy Paper.

DHSS (1983b). Health Service Development. Care in the Community and Joint Finance, Circular HC(83)6/LAC(83)5.

Richie J, Keegan J & Bosanquet N (1983). Housing for mentally ill and mentally handicapped people, Department of the Environment, HMSO.

Dick D H (1983). The Components of a Comprehensive Psychiatric Service, unpublished, available from King's Fund Centre.

MIND (1983). Common Concern. MIND, London.

Reed J L (1983). The DHSS Mental Illness Policy Paper: A Personal View, Bulletin of the Royal College of Psychiatrists, July.

PART ONE

THE IDEAS AND POLICIES BEHIND THE DEVELOPMENT OF COMPREHENSIVE LOCAL SERVICES

The chapters in the first part of this book investigate some of the theoretical debate and ideas from which present policies and practice derive. The first chapter, from the paper delivered to the conference by Lord Trefgarne, traces the history of government policies on mental health since 1972 and indicates some of the steps that are being taken to encourage progress in developing local services further. Authoritative comment is made by Professor Cawley, one of the instigators of an earlier move, a decade ago, towards locally-based services for mental illness.

The chapters which follow take up some of the points raised by Lord Trefgarne and Professor Cawley, and have been prepared from seminars given to the conference. Each of the authors has written about topics falling directly within his or her normal day-to-day activities or study. The chapters thus all reflect recent experience of the principles underlying the move towards comprehensive local psychiatric services.

Subjects selected for detailed treatment are information for psychiatric services; training for community psychiatry; ethical issues; sociological contributions to the debate; and the stigma associated with mental illness.

Chapter One

DEVELOPMENTS IN COMMUNITY PSYCHIATRY: A CENTRAL VIEW

Lord Trefgarne

Successive governments have subscribed to the policy
of caring for the mentally ill as an integral part
of society and not as a race apart. This is to me a
humane philosophy with which few members of that
society would disagree; although I am aware that
there are criticisms of the practical effects it can
sometimes have. The ten years that have elapsed
since ideas on a comprehensive district psychiatric
service were set down in **Policy for Action** (Cawley &
McLachlan 1973) have been eventful. This publication
was followed in 1975 by the White Paper, **Better
Services for the Mentally Ill** (DHSS 1975). It was as
clear then as it is now that it would take a good
deal of time to move away from a service based in
large, isolated hospitals.

In the years that have passed we have seen
large reductions in the numbers of beds occupied by
these patients - from over 100,000 in the early
1970s to 73,000 in 1980. Over the same period there
have been significant increases in the numbers of
residential and day centre places and the number of
day hospital places has more than doubled. There are
now about 160 psychiatric units in general
hospitals, although about half of them are quite
small.

Statistics can of course be misleading. For
instance, if I were to state that between 1973 and
1980 the number of local authority day centre places
increased by over one third, I imagine that people
would be impressed. If I then went on to state that
the actual number of new places this increase
represented was less than 200 a year, on average,
then the impact might be diminished.

Let me say two important things, therefore, on
the dangers of measuring progress only by the use of
official statistics. Firstly, they can be

misleading. They can, amongst other things, mask the
uneven progress that is being made in different
parts of the country. Second, they are incomplete.
For instance not all local authorities send in
returns and old figures have to be extrapolated.
Furthermore some important areas of provision, such
as group homes, are not always included.

However, it is still fair to say that a lot of
progress has been made and, although much remains to
be done, the basic principles we are following
remain the same. Various aspects of the policy have
developed at different paces and, along the way, the
emphasis may have changed - for example we have seen
a rapid development of community psychiatric nursing
services. All the same, the course we are steering
has not changed and I think it is still the right
one.

The policy we advocate and our commitment to it
were reaffirmed when we issued our handbook entitled
Care in Action (DHSS 1981a). We stated then that we
regarded the creation of local psychiatric services
in districts with few local provisions as an urgent
priority. We also said that there was a real need to
do away with those mental hospitals which will never
be well placed to provide a local service. We added,
'Such closures should provide a source of staff,
capital, and revenue to support the development of
the new pattern of health services for the mentally
ill, and perhaps help support the development of
services provided by local authorities.' I shall
describe below our 'Care in the Community' (see DHSS
1981b, 1983) initiative which again reflects our
consciousness of the needs of the new services. But
first as regards the old services, we are conscious
of the recommendations made by the Nodder Report in
1980 on how these hospitals ought best to be managed
and organised and how the process of change can best
be handled. This is not an easy policy and I am
aware of the very real anxieties that some people
feel about the prospects for discharged patients.
There are fears that if we push ahead too quickly
with closures then former patients will find
themselves back in a community which is not ready to
receive them. Of course, such fears are
understandable. Even though we have only closed
three hospitals in the 21 years that have elapsed
since the policy was first unfolded, the number of
inpatients has halved. But I am sure that the great
majority of patients who have come into the world
outside have benefited from this policy. This is
thanks to all the hard work done by health and local

authorities and voluntary organisations. These people now enjoy a less restricted, more dignified and altogether more satisfying life than they did in hospital. Provided we all continue to work together I am sure that the prospects for those still to be discharged are every bit as good.

This takes me on to the present status of the services. As I said, the aim is for each health district to have its own comprehensive psychiatric service which would include a psychiatric department in a district general hospital, with an assessment ward for elderly patients, day hospitals, local authority day and residential care, NHS continuing care and accommodation, for the elderly at least, community psychiatric nursing services and fieldwork support by the local authority and voluntary bodies. The psychiatric department in the district general hospital is becoming the focus of the local psychiatric service and the number of beds required in such a department for acute adult psychiatry — and therefore the size and nature of the department itself — is a subject of current debate and evaluation.

Two contributions to this debate are the paper produced by an official in my department's Operational Research Unit and the setting up of the Bed Usage Working Party by the Royal College of Psychiatrists. We have moved away from the idea of norms but if the Working Party can identify the factors which determine bed usage this will benefit anyone planning services in the future.

Important as it is to provide the right facilities and the right number of beds, the other ingredients such as joint planning, collaboration and multidisciplinary team work, are just as essential if a good, effective service is to be provided. I hope that these factors are well understood, and acted upon by all involved in the planning of services. There seems to be a growing feeling that communication and collaboration are key issues in the new pattern of psychiatric services — the issues that make or break it. Doctors, nurses, psychologists and social workers are increasingly developing services which link with or form part of community-based walk-in centres, crisis intervention services and community psychiatric nursing. These links also have the effect of stimulating developments in the community itself and this is especially true in the case of services which aim to intervene early on to reduce the risk of mental illness or to avoid its recurrence. I find these

developments imaginative and interesting - indeed
the Community Psychiatry Research Unit itself, at
Hackney Hospital, is one of them and a valuable
example it is. While we are doing this, however, we
must not lose sight of the problems of individuals
in the community who require longer-term care. The
people I have in mind are the elderly severely
mentally infirm, the patients who are difficult to
manage, and the 'new' long-stay patients.

My ministerial colleagues and I place great
emphasis on the development of services for elderly
people with psychiatric disorders. Without a really
effective service for this group, no local
psychiatric development can call itself comprehensive.

The most important of current developments
concerns our plans for the elderly. I have space to
give only a brief account but this will help to fill
out the monetary statement in the House of Commons
mentioned in the newspapers. First, the Health
Advisory Service has been carrying out a special
initiative in this field for the last couple of
years or so. This has culminated in a document which
Dr Dick has sent to every district to help them
develop their services (Health Advisory Service
1982).

My colleagues and I decided to take some
special steps to encourage the implementation of its
recommendations. Norman Fowler has coaxed a little
extra money out of the Chancellor and we are using
this £6 million to create 'demonstration development
districts' - we hope there will be one to each
region. We hope that these extra funds will enable
regional health authorities to build up a vigorous
strategy for ensuring the development of a proper,
comprehensive range of psychiatric services for the
elderly in every district. Local authority services
will need building up too, with the help of joint
finances. Successful candidates for 'demonstration
districts' will be those where health and local
authorities are really working together.

There have also been initiatives regarding the
problem of providing places in the new pattern of
services for those patients who are difficult to
manage. An important landmark was the Royal College
of Psychiatrists' report on secure facilities for
psychiatric patients (RCPsych 1980). My officials
are holding a series of meetings with regional
health authorities to discuss how problems can be
best resolved and it is intended to hold a
conference in 1983 involving all regions and those

professionals most concerned with the subject to seek a way forward.

The 'new' long-stay patients and their needs seem less clear: the picture varies from one district to another. The 1975 White Paper explained the thinking that lay behind the suggested hospital hostel; and research projects by Professor Wing and others are evaluating the work of such hostels.

We are most interested in links between primary health care and the specialist psychiatric services and the extent to which these are developing. To explore these relationships my officials will be arranging a gathering of interested persons some time in 1983 to discuss the research findings on the issues involved.

My Department is spending more than a million pounds this year on research in the mental illness field. The largest project is the one at Worcester. There we have spent a considerable sum of money over the last few years in helping the health authority and the local authority to develop the pattern of psychiatric services. We are now beginning to get results that can be evaluated and which can provide evidence about how different ways of doing things can affect what professionals can achieve.

Having thus moved back from the needs of individuals to the provision of services generally, I shall now briefly discuss our 'Care in the Community' initiative. There is nothing very different or new about the sentiments it embodies: the policy is still the same - that is, to move out of hospital those people who do not really need to be there. What we are trying to do is to make it easier to achieve that objective. We are going to make three administrative changes: the existing joint finance arrangements will be made more flexible; health authorities will be able to make continuing annual payments for as long as necessary for people moving into community care; £15 million of joint finance money is centrally reserved over the next five years to promote a programme of pilot projects. We do need some legislative changes. I therefore introduced into the House of Lords a Bill to extend joint finance to education for disabled people, including the mentally ill, and to housing, both important features of community care.

The Department places a high value on experiments and innovation in service provision by statutory and voluntary bodies. None of us can pretend that we have all the answers on how best to provide a service for the mentally ill in the

community and we must all remain receptive towards
novel and different approaches. Let me commend to
you in passing the idea of enrolling your local
services for the 'Good Practices in Mental Health'
project, directed by Mrs Morgan and mentioned in
other chapters of this book.

We also recognise the importance of local
community effort and informal care. Funds have been
made available through the 'Opportunities for
Volunteering' scheme to enable some unemployed
people who feel they could make a worthwhile
personal contribution to play a part as volunteers.
Individual local projects and the administration of
the scheme are being handled entirely within the
voluntary sector.

Finally I should like to enumerate six ways in
which we, centrally, can help to ensure that
psychiatric services get their fair share in the
future and that resources develop along the lines
spelt out in the 1975 White Paper. Firstly, the fact
that services for the mentally ill are a ministerial
priority should help. This was made clear in **Care in
Action** and I reaffirm it here. Second, Norman Fowler
has instituted a programme of annual reviews with
each regional health authority chairman to consider
the region's plans. This is an opportunity for the
Department to monitor the progress of planned
services for the mentally ill and in fact mental
health is the one area that has been covered in
every review so far. Third, we have now issued a
circular initiating action on our 'Care in the
Community' initiative (DHSS 1983). Fourth, my
Department hopes to issue further guidance on day
care for the mentally ill following the exercise
instigated by my predecessor, Sir George Young. This
will pull together the accumulated knowledge in the
country on the state of the art and provide useful
information to those responsible for planning the
provision of such services. Fifth, the 1983 Mental
Health Act recently became law, as you know, and is
a significant step forward in improving the legal
position of the mentally disordered in many
different ways. One important point to note in
relation to the care of detained patients is that
tribunals are to be given increased flexibility to
recommend options other than discharge. They will in
future be able to recommend discharge at a future
date (thus allowing arrangements to be made for
looking after the patient in the community) or
recommend that the patient be transferred to another
hospital or be given leave of absence. This should

make it easier to ensure satisfactory arrangements
are made to provide care in the most suitable place
- whether in the community or in another hospital.
Sixth, improvements in services are influenced as
much by what local professionals do as by what the
Department says. After all, departmental guidance is
based on a consensus of what is thought to be good
practice and if the planners of services, the
providers of resources and the practitioners are to
be influenced for the good it calls for the combined
efforts of us all. Changing the attitudes of all
those involved in providing services for the
mentally ill is a major task. Professionals are very
much influenced by professionals. This is why I as
an amateur am pleased to launch your professional
debates and discussions. These are important in
maintaining the momentum for changes and improvements.

The development of comprehensive district
psychiatric services is the target for us all. We
are regarded as pioneers by those in other
countries: let us aspire to continue to lead the
way.

DISCUSSION AND COMMENTS

R H Cawley

Something which starts out from the most miserable
beginnings, if it is really good, can turn out well.
But it takes time to learn how to meet commitments,
how to use one's assets, to learn that money helps
but is not everything and that exercise of the brain
can be productive when money is a bit short. The
question we should be asking is how far along the
line - the scale from disregarded impoverishment to
the state ultimately to be desired - have the
psychiatric services travelled?

The first part of this book is being devoted to
ideas and policies behind the development of
district services, and Lord Trefgarne has given us
the central view. Let me say a little about the
background view, and the two-way relationship
between principles and practice; especially in areas
of progress over the last ten years. Firstly, within
medicine, psychiatry is now clearly recognised as a

major specialty, and within medicine it shares much common ground with general practice. A good deal of progress has been made in recognising this and in improving liaison. But psychiatry has an equally important and very substantial part of its being outside medicine. This has come clearly to light in recent years. This part of it, outside medicine as well as inside medicine, is what makes it such a fascinating and important subject. No one discipline in psychiatry can claim exclusiveness. It depends for its knowledge on many sciences, basic sciences (biology and psychology), applied social studies and clinical medical sciences. In academic terms it is perhaps the busiest junction in the world. Lord Trefgarne mentioned public attitudes and pro-fessional attitudes. These have advanced, if not to the state of what is ultimately to be desired, at least some steps along the road. If psychiatry is now recognised to be a multidisciplinary affair, then the practice of psychiatry must be multi-professional, depending on the skills of many disciplines. Inexorable logic points to the multi-professional team as the most effective instrument at all stages in the process of planning and execution of services and it is worth noting that it is logic and not dogma that urges the importance of seeing psychiatric practice as a multi-professional endeavour.

What has clearly emerged also over the years is that the hierarchies, the chains of command and responsibility, are within rather than between, professional groups. This principle underlines the importance of communication; the efforts of different professional groups must be co-ordinated and harmonised, both in planning services, and in the management of individual clients. A psychiatric team, for all its skill and power, is dependent upon a lot of other people, and amongst these housing is crucial. It is not now possible to contemplate a good district psychiatric service which does not have the active interest and support of its district housing department and of housing associations.

In the present state of the service, local variation and experiment is of the essence: clients, problems and professional attitudes vary, and local social and demographic variables always influence what can be done and what is desirable. My view on several of these counts is a favourable one: the last ten years have brought us quite a way along the scale. Perhaps we should now have less moaning about the >Cinderella' service, and there are good reasons for dropping the notion. Not surprisingly, there are a few lapses from time to time, and I see two cardinal errors of which we may all be guilty now and then. The first mistake is the notion that community care is a convenient way of combining progress with the opportunity for economising. The second is the idea that all problems in the service are attributable to lack of money or that all problems would be resolved by having more money.

There remain other important questions; a central one is how we can help each other. Lord Trefgarne has indicated that services for the mentally ill are a ministerial priority. How can we turn this to advantage? What initiatives and liaison are needed from the DHSS, with its central role? What might be provided from the regions? One of the things that taxes me from time to time is how to introduce, locally, some innovation that has been pioneered somewhere else. How can we apply the findings of research? The problem often is not in basic health services research but in finding the support and funding to take the results of research already done and to test and modify to suit local circumstances. It is usually rather difficult to find a pocket for this sort of health service development, since it falls a bit between what ought to be the routine service and what is strictly health service research.

Another point along a similar line: what are the pros and cons of functional budgeting for a district? What are the local realities of joint planning between the health district and the local authority? How can professional organisations and the voluntary bodies help each other and reinforce each others efforts? How can we help patients or clients to retain as much autonomy as possible without becoming isolated? How can we enable them to retain elements of choice in their lives?

Finally I am pleased to see that there is to be some review of information systems. There is an urgent need for data at all levels and, of course, all the time the service is operating in all its complexity, data is being generated but tends to be lost. There is a need for regular information about the work of professionals, about various schemes, about methods of co-ordination, and about particular services and individual clients. It is important also to recall that we must not fail to capitalise on the power of modern information and technology, to support and inform and assist the human factor.

REFERENCES

Cawley R H & McLachlan G (eds) (1973). <u>Policy for Action</u>. A Symposium on the Planning of a Comprehensive District Psychiatric Service. OUP, London.

DHSS (1975). <u>Better Services for the Mentally Ill</u>. Cmnd 6233, HMSO.

DHSS (1981a). <u>Care in Action</u>. HMSO.

DHSS (1981b). <u>Care in the Community</u>. A Consultative Document on Moving Resources for Care in England. Circular HC(81)9/LAC(81)5.

DHSS (1983). <u>Health Service Development. Care in the Community and Joint Finance</u>. Circular HC(83)6/LAC(83)5.

Health Advisory Service (1982). <u>The Rising Tide</u>. Developing Services for Mental Illness in Old Age. NHS; HAS.

Royal College of Psychiatrists (1980). <u>Secure Facilities for Psychiatric Patients. A Comprehensive Policy</u>. Unpublished.

Chapter Two

INFORMATION FOR PSYCHIATRIC SERVICES

Neil Zammett and Jill Sternfeld

The changes which are currently taking place in psychiatric services in this country rely to a great extent on having adequate and up-to-date information for planning and monitoring. A well-designed, flexible information system is especially important when a comprehensive service is made up of a number of different elements, supplied by several different authorities. If services have to be planned without the benefit of a good information and research base, it is more likely that there will be overlapping facilities in some areas and gaps in others, than it is that supply and demand will coincide. Information available at present is inadequate in many ways to satisfy the demands that will be made in the future. This chapter gives a brief summary of what is collected regularly, notes some of the deficiencies and makes some suggestions about the important considerations for improving the information base for psychiatric services.

Statistics about mental illness come from three standard returns: the SH3, the SBH112 and the HMR1, the latter forming the basis of the Mental Health Enquiry (MHE). The DHSS publishes two series of reports containing standard tables together with useful lists of definitions and notes on the record forms (DHSS various dates). The Welsh Office produces similar information for hospitals in Wales. Each regional health authority collects, processes and analyses the data from the standard forms filled in for each hospital. The information acquired in this way is used for its own planning purposes, often involving forecasting of patient numbers and such things as bed usage for ten or twenty years ahead, and also for dissemination to the constituent health districts for their own planning and monitoring purposes.

A REGIONAL VIEW OF INFORMATION

The routine manual systems which are used for statistics such as those from the SH3, giving, for example, daily bed occupancy, have a number of drawbacks. Most importantly, they are generalised systems, designed to provide information for and about the acute services, and, as such, are not adaptable for community-oriented services where the emphasis is not on actual beds. These routine systems do not convey much about the different patient groups and sub-groups either as analysed now, or potentially.

The standard statistical systems as applied to mental illness are deficient in a number of ways:

- most systems assume that patients form a homogeneous group, whereas with mental illness there are wide ranges to consider.
- the Mental Health Enquiry, which is the only computerised system at the moment, concentrates exclusively on admissions and discharges, saying nothing about the resident populations of the large psychiatric hospitals nor about the increasing numbers of patients treated on a day or outpatient basis.
- systems are inaccessible to most professionals at their place of work, and information is not very easily available at regional offices. To acquire information someone from the computing department has to extract the data; this means that requirements have to be exactly specified in advance and that there is a time-lag.

There are several more general points to take into consideration. Firstly, for the sort of service which is envisaged for mental illness in the future it is vital that we are able to study the dynamic aspects of both the supply and use made of services. The present information systems provide only static views, making it virtually impossible to assess flows, particularly where specific patient categories, say psychogeriatric patients, or 'old' long-stay, are concerned. We should, perhaps, be considering whether there is a case for different forms of information systems for separate categories of patient.

A second point concerns the relationships between the large hospital (where there is one) and the smaller local unit(s). This is an area where, operationally, it is most important to have comparable information about, for instance, the flows of patients, length of stay, and patient characteristics. However, there are also bound to be types of information needed in local units – assuming that they cater more for the acute phases of mental illness – which are not so important for the larger hospitals. At the moment there are no ways, using the standard systems, of linking information for individual patients or groups of patients as they move between or through different elements of a comprehensive service.

To be successful in satisfying the needs of planners and practitioners, any system, as well as allowing dynamic analysis rather than simply that of static resources, must also be accessible to the people who use it and must interact with the environment in which they are working. The HMR1, as an example, is filled in for every patient who is discharged from hospital. The office clerk who fills in the form will rarely see any of the information produced from all the forms and may have no idea of any of the uses to which the data are put. Indeed, consultant psychiatrists may have an equally vague idea of the uses to which information about their patients is put. Such a system is hardly likely to encourage accuracy and is, in practice, not well run. It does illustrate the need for direct feedback and for better interaction.

Present systems are, on the whole, quite inflexible, suffering from the blight of standardisation. Professionally, a 'standard' system, using a number of standard forms and methods of analysis, is easier and more cost-effective to design than a custom-built one. However, it will be more difficult to implement and will rarely be satisfactory for the user. We have to recognise that the types of information needed at regional level are not able to satisfy the needs of planners at district level; information needed for stategic, long-term planning will not enable an administrator or consultant to redeploy current staff or change the balance of elements of a service within one unit.

Finally, there are large areas where there is no satisfactory information at all, despite the seemingly regular collection of many items of data. The decline in inpatient numbers is probably the single most important feature of mental illness services at the present time, yet, apart from the SH3, which shows a general decline in bed occupancy, there is no statistical system which can demonstrate

the ways in which the composition of the population
is changing. This situation has been identified, and
described from survey work, for a long time, but no
information system has been able to respond in order
to monitor the detailed characteristics of change on
a national basis.

To summarise, the important points for improving the information base, from a regional
viewpoint, are accessibility of information for the
user, relevance and a degree of interaction, particular concentration on the identification and
description of key areas of change and a
consideration of the advantages and disadvantages of
a central, standardised system.

SOURCES OF INFORMATION

Within each district information of various kinds is
needed for the planning and monitoring of
psychiatric services. In particular, information is
needed about

- the population and its needs
- demands made by that population
- resources which are provided
- how these resources are used
- the outcome of how resources are used

Information about a range of demographic and
socio-economic characteristics of the population of
a district, or smaller areas within a district, is
available from the decennial Census of Population,
and forms a background to much planning. Some items,
such as age and sex structure, are amended and
projected on an annual basis by various authorities.
Information about need is less easily come by,
although some forms of mortality may be used as a
proxy for psychiatric morbidity, and other aspects
of morbidity can be inferred from the reported use
of the services which are provided. The Mental
Health Enquiry, restricted to inpatients in
psychiatric hospitals and units (and completed only
on discharge), is the only source of diagnostic
information. All inferences that we might make about
need as related to diagnosis are, in consequence,
influenced by the admissions and discharge policies
reflected in the HMR1 returns from which the MHE is
prepared.

The following notes give an indication of the
sources of information which might be utilised and

the gaps, but does not enter into discussion of the accuracy or completeness of the available data.

Inpatients. The numbers of available beds, occupied beds and discharges are produced annually from the SH3. The form SBH112 provides details on staffing – medical, nursing and therapists. This form also records data on the numbers of patients participating in activities such as outside employment, and on patient amenities, such as personal cupboard space. The main source of information about inpatients is the MHE which has details of each admission and discharge. These data are at present analysed nationally, by computer, by the Office of Population Censuses and Surveys. In addition to a national report, OPCS produces standard computer printout for each of the regions, analysed by district. Each region also has a tape containing all the data from which specially requested tabulations could be computed, though not all regions take advantage of this.

Outpatients. SH3 records the numbers of sessions, new patients and day patients.

Day patients. Attendances are recorded on SH3. Age, by attendance on one day is available from SBH112.

Primary and community care. As far as the community psychiatric nurses are concerned, information is available about staff complements but not about what they do. Nothing is known (officially) about what occurs in general practice, although it may be possible to obtain some information in an indirect fashion by analysing information about the prescription of psychotropic drugs.

    There are considerable gaps and innumerable problems with the system as it is arranged at present, these problems pervade all the categories mentioned above. The major problems are:

    1. There is always a time-lag of several years
       between the collection of data and its becoming
       available for use, even by professionals. The
       time-lag for research workers and others is
       even greater.
    2. Information suffers greatly from the
       impossibility of linking the different parts of
       the service. For example, it is possible, for
       each year, to say how many new outpatients

there are, and how many day hospital patients attend; it is not possible to identify how many are common to both. A further anomaly exists when, as is commonly the case, a patient has to be re-referred after a six-month period with no contact with the psychiatric service. It is possible for one person to appear twice as a 'new' patient and thus wreak havoc on any attempts that might be made to assess need from the data relating to attendances. With this system it is not possible, ever, to analyse information about the service with the patient, the consumer, as the subject. The pattern of care as provided to individuals, can never be established. This implies that, in practice, it is not possible to arrive at costs (either financial or social), over the many years of chronic mental illness, of alternative forms of care; a problem which bedevils many research projects - and practical planning exercises.

3. As mentioned earlier in this chapter, in the context of regional planning, there is increasing momentum for community-oriented services, backed (unfortunately) by information bases geared to totally outdated (in relation to psychiatric care, certainly) styles of treatment which tend to recognise only inpatient care as worthy of note.

4. The outcome of any form of treatment or care is virtually unknown except in a most anecdotal sense.

The problems surrounding the provision of information for the wide variety of needs which are familiar to most planners and practitioners are pretty well recognised. The DHSS set up a joint steering group to consider all aspects of information for the NHS under the chairmanship of Mrs Edith Korner (DHSS 1983). This group has made a number of recommendations which are relevant to the collection and dissemination of information for hospital psychiatric services. Previously, an internal review in the DHSS had suggested that the regional health authorities should themselves take over responsibility for the analysis and further dissemination of the MHE information. It was, incidentally, suggested that the collection of data which could be attributed to a named individual be discontinued. This is an issue with important, often misunderstood, implications, and one on which expert debate and decision is urgently required.

In summary, the Korner recommendations, insofar
as they apply to psychiatric services, are:

1. There should no longer be a separate
   computerised inpatient system for psychiatric
   services, but the same system should cover
   psychiatric, non-psychiatric and maternity
   patients. Data should be analysed by the
   regional health authorities.
2. There should be an annual census of patients
   who have been resident in hospitals for one
   year or more, primarily to determine whether
   such patients are appropriately placed.
3. Information relating to the administering of
   electroconvulsive therapy (ECT) should be recorded in the census and on discharge of
   patients.

The really important issue, that of linking
different parts of a psychiatric service, for
dynamic analysis of the provision and use of a
service which is used by a very wide spectrum of the
country's population, was not tackled by the
Steering Group.

From the point of view of a District
Information Officer, responsible for providing
information for district (and lower level) planning
and monitoring over the whole range of health
services, the following points are of most immediate
relevance: firstly, to improve the access and
usefulness of existing data systems; secondly, to
have local systems where a case can be made for
them; thirdly, to reduce the reliance on 'standard'
systems and make more use of properly conducted
surveys; and to encourage (and finance?) psychiatric
service registers for each district.

As may be apparent from the contents of this
chapter, the outlook for information for psychiatric
services is fraught with difficulties, especially in
the context of potentially radical changes in the
style of delivery of services, which, with the
benefit of hindsight, we might come to recognise as
being of importance comparable to the introduction
of long-acting anti-psychotic medication (although
with a much more protracted time-span). It is not
surprising that many worthy attempts to clarify the
relationships between demand and supply of services
falter on the seemingly simple questions of who does
what, to whom, where, how often, and with what
result.

REFERENCES

DHSS (various years). In-patient Statistics from the
    Mental Health Enquiry for England. Statistical and
    Research Report Series, HMSO.
DHSS (various years). Facilities and services of
    mental illness and mental handicap hospitals in
    England. Statistical and Research Report Series,
    HMSO.
DHSS (1983). Health Services Information. First
    Report to the Secretary of State by the Steering
    Group (Chairman, Mrs E Korner), HMSO.

Chapter Three

TRAINING IN COMMUNITY PSYCHIATRY

Sam Baxter

In recent years a new sub-specialty of community psychiatry has developed (Freeman 1983). It is a difficult specialty to define, since it does not encompass any particular group of patients such as those who have been in contact with the courts or need psychotherapy, nor does it apply to a particular age group such as children or the elderly. There are suggestions that community psychiatrists differ from more 'ordinary' psychiatrists in that they have greater expertise in dealing with the boundaries between health and social services, that they have training in mental health planning and even that they are better at liaising with primary care teams and community psychiatric nurses. They might also be concerned more with prevention of illness by working, for instance, in the bereavement service, with volunteers or with a crisis intervention team.

In order to further our ideas about ways of training psychiatrists to work in a community-oriented service, we should first look at the needs of the mentally ill in any geographical area, and at what services will be needed now and in the future to serve them best. The core work of any catchment area-based psychiatric service is the care of those people who are chronically ill. Most people suffering from chronic, long-term disabilities will not be very ill all the time; nevertheless they require continuing surveillance and care. Previously this care was provided in hospital, but increasingly such patients are being cared for in the community, i.e. they do not <u>live</u> in hospital. Hence the catchment area psychiatrist is responsible for devising and running, in consultation with social services, nursing, volunteers, and other colleagues, a service which reduces the emphasis on

hospitalisation and increases the emphasis on
support during crises for people in their own homes,
in hostels or other accommodation. It is not
realistic to suppose that this can be done by a
psychiatrist sitting in a hospital, even a hospital
within the community. Psychiatrists must learn to
seek more active involvement outside hospitals, by
going out to meet social workers, by visiting
hostels, and by providing back-up services for other
professionals working with the mentally ill. This is
hardly a new idea, yet it is not reflected adequately in the training which we give to psychiatrists.

Psychiatrists are initially trained as doctors.
To become a doctor means achieving high grades at
'A' level, usually in science subjects, and then
studying for five or six years at a university.
Approximately two years are spent in learning about
the structure and functioning of the body, and three
years studying patients and their illnesses and
possible cures. Doctors are trained in the diagnosis
and treatment of disease according to a model which
has little room for the idea that illness might be
rooted in a social, psychological or cultural
context. The model is seen as universal in that once
you have trained to be a doctor in one part of the
world, you might have to learn about a few different
diseases if you go elsewhere, but the model will
remain the same. In recent years there has been
concern that this process has gone too far, so it is
remedied by a few lectures in sociology or about
'the family', which are treated as another
specialist field like pathology or psychiatry.
Students will probably leave medical school with
some theoretical idea that social factors may have
some relevance to the causation of ill health, but
they will probably not see this as being relevant to
their way of treating disease. They will know little
about the life styles of their prospective patients,
and even less about the NHS for which they will work
and which provides the basic structure of health
care in this country. They will know nothing about
the politics of the delivery of health care.

After qualifying in medicine, a mandatory year
is spent practising medicine and surgery under close
supervision in a hospital. The doctor is then free
to choose which special branch of medicine to
follow, and it is common to spend another year or
more in general hospital work. Some specialties are
very much more popular than others; psychiatry is
one of the less popular ones. This reflects the

continuing prejudice against the mentally ill and
low status compared with surgeons and physicians.
Students commonly view psychiatry as being
unscientific and lacking in precision in the ideas
it uses. Trainees in psychiatry will probably spend
their first year or so working primarily with
inpatients, being taught to take detailed histories
from their patients and also their families and
other relevant people - in the context of the
hospital ward. The theory, apparently, is that until
a trainee has actually learned to identify and treat
psychiatric diseases, he is not safe to be let out
into the wider world of psychiatric practice. By
working in the ward he will be protected from any
great mistakes by the fact that the patients are
being looked after in a closed environment and there
will be competent nurses and other colleagues to
oversee his work.

A psychiatrist will spend three years as a
junior trainee, and at this stage, even in theory,
has only limited experience of psychiatry in a
setting beyond the hospital. A further three or four
years will normally be spent as a senior registrar
trainee, and it is at this stage that the Royal
College of Psychiatrists expects that specialist
knowledge of 'community psychiatry' should be
acquired. There are only five full-time posts in
community psychiatry in England and Wales, though
there are other posts which offer part-time
experience. Such posts are often based in a day
hospital and are certainly likely to afford some
experience of what goes on outside the hospital. It
is still seen as a specialist activity which is
tacked on to the core problem of hospital-based management of psychiatric illness (see RCPsych 1980,
Wing & Morris 1981). One disadvantage, for the
would-be community psychiatrist is that not all
doctors who become consultant psychiatrists will
have had any training themselves in these wider
aspects of psychiatric care. It continues to be
possible to become a consultant without having any
significant amount of experience outside a hospital
setting. For many consultants hospital and community
remain separate entities as far as treatment is
concerned.

Probably the most fundamental aspect of
training in psychiatry is the treatment and management of mentally ill people in the context of the
community within which they become ill, and of the
families who will have the major role in caring for
them. Training must involve learning about the

resources available for treating and supporting patients and families, of which the inpatient unit will be only one, albeit the most highly staffed. Of course, all psychiatrists must be competent to take adequate histories and diagnose psychiatric illness and know the appropriate medical treatments, but these skills should be regarded as only part of the wider management of patients in terms of the total resources available. Community psychiatry cannot be continue to be treated as a separate sub-specialty, since for the forseeable future all psychiatric services will incorporate treatment and long-term support to patients who spend only short periods within the hospital itself. We can only train psychiatrists to take this wider view by allowing our trainees more autonomy and more supervision.

Virtually unnoticed, the same trainee psychiatrists will be covering emergencies that turn up in the casualty department. In two unpublished surveys which I carried out, some years apart, at Hackney Hospital and at Charing Cross Hospital, I discovered that half of all new patients seen in the psychiatric unit were being seen, mostly unsupervised, by trainee psychiatrists in the Accident and Emergency Department. The disease model of lengthy, leisurely history-taking, differential diagnoses, and treatment plans, is rarely relevant to these patients who present at various levels of crisis of which psychiatric illness, its diagnosis and treatment, is only part. They need help from a variety of sources, of which the inpatient unit is only one, though frequently the only one of which the trainee is aware. Since junior psychiatrists are already running the emergency psychiatric service in most parts of the country, usually relatively unsupervised, then the step might not appear so large. They should also be going out to make home assessments, visiting GP surgeries and social services offices, following their patients through hostels and day centres, meeting housing workers and employers. There must be acknowledgement by them and their consultants that they will have to take and implement some decisions without prior detailed discussion with the consultant. The multi-professional organisation of the service should enable psychiatrists to get advice and assistance making it unnecessary for decisions to be taken in isolation. They (and we) must not fear leaving the comforting confines of the ward for the real world which is where most psychiatrically ill people spend most of their lives.

My experience is that trainee psychiatrists enjoy working in a community-oriented setting, especially having relative autonomy, as a psychiatrist, in work with other professionals. Once they are confident that it is safe to leave the ward they soon function effectively, providing a useful service and learning a wide range of skills. The problem lies with their superiors: how can we persuade them to interest their trainees in the community?

REFERENCES

Freeman H (1983). Concepts of Community Psychiatry. British Journal of Hospital Medicine, 30, 90-96.
Royal College of Psychiatrists (1980). Psychiatric Rehabilitation in the 1980s. RCPsych, London.
Wing J K & Morris B (eds) (1981). Handbook of Psychiatric Rehabilitation Practice. OUP, London.

Chapter Four

ETHICAL ISSUES IN COMMUNITY-BASED PSYCHIATRY

Ian E Thompson

SUMMARY

An analysis of the ethical basis of the traditional caring professions reveals that there are three fundamental values which are basic to their practice:

1. Respect for persons. This refers to the commitment to treat people as ends rather than as means, to protect the dignity of individuals, and to respect their personal rights.
2. Justice. This is the requirement of universal fairness, that people should be treated equally, without discrimination, while protecting the common good.
3. Beneficence. This is the recognition of a responsibility to do good rather than harm to others, accepting the duty to care for the vulnerable on the basis that one might at some time be in need of care oneself.

This chapter examines a range of ethical issues related to the provision of a community-oriented service in psychiatry, in the light of these three values and ethical principles derived from them.

ETHICAL VALUES IN THE CARING PROFESSIONS

The fundamental values of respect for persons, justice and beneficence have a wide applicaton in virtually all known ethical systems - different systems giving particular weight of emphasis to one or the other or all three - but they are also of particular relevance to the practice of the caring professions.

Respect for persons is perhaps the most

fundamental and is presupposed by the other two. The principle of personhood as an end in itself, as something valuable and to be protected, underlies our concepts of justice and the duty to care. Justice is the value which expresses the demand that we extend respect for persons to all persons equally, the principle that our ethical rules should be universally applicable. However, this very demand for universal justice or pursuit of the common good may set limits to individual rights in order to protect the rights of others. Because there are inherent inequalities between people and there may be a need to protect the rights of the weak against the strong, there is a need for beneficence - a recognition of the duty to care, based on the principle of reciprocity, namely, that we should do for others what we hope they would do for us if we were unable to defend our own interests.

In the development of community-based services, both statutory and voluntary, for the mentally disordered, these values have great importance as guides to good practice.

Respect for persons means treating people as persons with rights. In general this means that professionals and those in a caring role have a responsibility to give people the right kind of information to enable them to make responsible choices for themselves. It means adopting an enabling rather than a controlling role so as to facilitate people's autonomy, and elicit their full potential to help themselves. It means not turning people into dependants medically or educationally. With respect to patients in particular it involves recognising that they have a right to know, a right to privacy (i.e. a right to the protection of their personal dignity and confidential disclosures), and a right to adequate care or treatment.

Justice, or non-discrimination, means both equality of opportunity for individuals and equality of outcome for groups. For individuals justice primarily means fairness, in particular non-discrimination on the basis of sex, race, class or religion, and not taking advantage of or neglecting those who are vulnerable by virtue of extreme youth, old age, handicap or mental disorder. However, the opportunities for self-fulfilment and self-determination of individuals might have to be restricted where the common good demands this, to facilitate more equal distribution of resources, or where others may be put at risk. The political dimensions of justice in terms of equality of outcome for groups has particular relevance to health care not only in making services acceptable and accessible to all groups in the population, but also by the exercise of political control and reverse discrimination to provide for the needs of the most vulnerable and needy groups. Justice at this level is not only concerned with rational planning of public health and the provision, for example, of a National Health Service, but demands adequate public consultation, consumer feedback and participation in the planning of services. In protecting the public from harm there may be a need for public health legislation or legal controls to sanction the compulsory hospitalisation and treatment of those who are dangerous to themselves or others by virtue of serious mental disorder. It also means providing adequate means for their rehabilitation and measures to ensure professional accountability.

   <u>Beneficence</u> relates most obviously to the duty of professionals or others to care for vulnerable individuals entrusted into their care - children, the elderly, incompetents or the mentally disordered - but it also relates to the responsibility of the professional to act as an advocate in the best interests of his clients - the role of advocacy and fiduciary responsibility go together. Secondly, it refers to the responsibility of the professional to share his knowledge and expertise for the benefit of the patient or client. Knowledge is power, and being kept in a state of ignorance may mean being kept in a state of powerlessness. Sharing knowledge is not just a matter of obtaining informed consent to treatment, but using the disclosure of relevant information as an aid to therapy and the progressive restoration of autonomy to the patient.

   Sharing expertise means using the best available skills and resources for the benefit of those needing help or therapy, remembering always that efficiency and competence are the kindest forms of care. Mere compassion is no substitute for properly tested procedures and objective testing of costs and benefits of various available procedures. Thirdly, beneficence relates to the educational and political responsibilities of professionals as persons enjoying public confidence for their service to the community. This includes the responsibilities of public office to educate individuals and inform public opinion about the needs of vulnerable individuals and groups, to pressure for the just distribution of resources and to ensure proper

standards of competence in the caring professions
through adequate education and training.

COMMUNITY PSYCHIATRY - IS IT REALLY BETTER THAN INSTITUTIONAL CARE?

The principles discussed above in very general terms
now need to be applied more specifically to attempts
to develop community-based approaches to psychiatry.
First, however, we need to ask some preliminary
questions. Why community psychiatry? Is is really
better than institutional care? Attempts to answer
these questions raise further questions about
fundamental values in health care and the relative
merits of different theoretical models for
understanding the phenomenon of mental disorder in
individuals and how they interact with their
families and society.

Doctors and social workers have a different
training and tend to construe social reality in
different ways according to the 'ideologies' of
their respective professions. The 'medical model' -
concerned as it is with diagnosis and therapeutic
intervention - results in a conceptualisation of
mental disorder predominantly in terms of 'mental
illness' and tends to focus on hospital-based
'treatment'. The 'social work model' - concerned
with the identification of vulnerable individuals or
families who are 'at risk' or 'problem cases' -
tends to conceptualise mental disorder in terms of
social deviance or reaction to stress and
environmental factors. It tends to offer either
individual counselling and support (including skills
training) or community initiatives aimed at
mobilising the skills and resources of groups to
help vulnerable individuals and to change the
environmental conditions. Within these two broad
groupings there are also varieties of specialist
approaches with their ardent advocates and
disciples.

In the first instance is the shift from
hospital to community a 'victory' for the 'social
work model' over the 'medical model'? Or, is it
rather a case of the medical profession abrogating
responsibility for a group of problem individuals
who were previusly thought to be candidates for
therapy but with whom the therapeutic approach has
failed and who are now being pushed back into the
community as the responsibility of social workers
and voluntary agencies?

Secondly, what are the relative costs and

benefits of the two approaches? Have these been
properly researched or is this just a change of
fashion with dubious scientific justification? Are
the two models incompatible, or are they not rather
complementary? What are the relative financial costs
of the two approaches and who carries the cost?
Which is the more efficient way of using
professional expertise and resources? Which approach
is more beneficial for 'patients', and least
burdensome to the family or community?

Thirdly, are there different consequences for
the treatment of acute or chronic cases in the
community? Should the community be bearing the
burden of care for the chronically 'ill'? For example, how do we balance the ill effects of institutionalisation with the ill effects of inadequate
community care, or the deskilling effects of long-
stay 'treatment' in hospital with chronic disability
in the community, or the benefits of asylum, albeit
dependency-inducing, with independence without
security or social support (Hawks 1975)?

ETHICAL ISSUES IN COMMUNITY PSYCHIATRY

Applying the three basic values to community
psychiatry we are driven to examine the following
issues:

1. Fundamental rights of patients or clients
   (Respect for Persons).
2. The scope and limits of professional duty
   (Beneficence).
3. Individual needs and community involvement and
   responsibility (Justice).

1. Respect for Persons and Patients' Rights

The rights of patients/clients are derived from and
related to the fundamental assumptions underlying
the contract established when a vulnerable person
entrusts himself into the care of another and the
carer accepts the duty to care: people seek help
under the duress of felt need, fear, pain or
distress. In that condition they are inherently
vulnerable and need to be protected. By entrusting
themselves into the care of another they make an act
of moral faith in the carer. By accepting the duty
to care the carer accepts 'fiduciary responsibility'
for the client. Fiduciary responsibility gives the
carer certain privileges and power over the client
which he may abuse but is expected to use 'in the
best interests' of the client. In view of the nature

of the implicit contract with the carer the client
has certain rights: the right to know, the right to
privacy and the right to treatment. The right to
know flows from the fact that the client exposes
himself to examination (physical, psychological and
social) on the assumption that the caring professional will in turn give him appropriate
information relative to the care and management of
his case. The right to privacy covers both confidentiality and respect for the dignity of the
client's person and relates to the vulnerability of
the client and the carer's undertaking to protect
his interests. The right to care and treatment is
related to the cause which brings the client to the
carer for help in the first place and the positive
right to be cared for is also balanced by the
negative right to refuse treatment.

Two general points need to be made about
rights. No rights are absolute, since the exercise
of his rights by one man may limit the rights of
another. Secondly, when dealing with mental disorder
major ambiguities enter into the discussion of the
rights of affected individuals, which relate to
their moral and legal status as moral agents, that
is whether they are competent to make responsible
moral decisions or not. In such cases professional
carers may acquire special responsibility to protect
the rights of mentally disordered clients.

The right to know. With mentally disordered
individuals there are not only problems about
whether patients should be told their diagnosis, but
whether they should give consent to treatment or be
given treatment whether they want it or not. Clearly
mentally disordered individuals and their families
have just as much entitlement as anyone else to be
informed of their rights. However we are becoming
aware that the extent to which individuals can
really exercise their rights within institutions may
be very limited whether or not they are 'ill', but
equally questions arise about the extent to which
treatment offered in the community is voluntary or
compulsory and how much relatives pressurise
patients into compliance. How far are people
constrained by social pressure to accept treatment
which they would be legally or morally entitled to
refuse? The right to know really means giving
patients information in a form and manner which
empowers them to make reasonably independent
choices.

Consent to treatment should be both informed

and voluntary. It is inherently difficult to satisfy
both these criteria in dealing with psychiatric
patients, whether in an institutional setting or the
community. Part of the difficulty relates to the
status of the patient, his competence or otherwise
to make decisions, but it also relates to the
vagueness of what counts as 'treatment' in
psychiatry - ranging from ECT and chemotherapy to
psychoanalysis, group therapy, occupational therapy,
and physiotherapy to nursing care and community
support (whether asked for or not). How much is
being consented to when consent is given, how much
is the patient entitled to refuse? An informal
patient can discharge himself from hospital if he
does not like what he is getting. Can he equally
easily refuse the visit from social worker or the
community psychiatric nurse to his home?
    Diagnosis in psychiatry has an ambiguous
significance for the patient in hospital, apart from
the notorious difficulty of defining clinically the
specific syndromes which characterise the great
variety of possible forms of human distress. On the
one hand medical diagnosis, in seeking other causes
for mental illness, relieves the patient of blame
and personal responsiblity for his condition and
legitimates his call upon medical services for care
and treatment. On the other hand, diagnosis can very
easily be seen as an instrument for legitimating
social control of deviant individuals or the mentally 'ill'. Diagnosis is, for the patient, both a
ticket to the privileges of the sick role and also
something which stigmatises him with the label of
mental illness. The loss of liberty and privacy
which submitting to social control of your 'illness'
entails, whether in the hospital or community, and
the disadvantages of being stigmatised, have to be
balanced against the rights of access which the sick
role gives you to medical and social resources. The
painful ambiguity of the status of being diagnosed
mentally ill is not lessened in a community setting
but may be worse without the protection which
hospital can give.

The right to privacy. This right is not so much
concerned with privacy in hospital wards or the
right to private medicine as with the patient's
right to the protection of his physical and psychological vulnerability, protection of his personal
dignity and respect for his confidences shared in
the process of consultation and treatment. A major
ethical issue in psychiatry is that of respect for

confidentiality. In the team management of patients a system of 'extended confidentiality' tends to operate, sometimes with the patient's knowledge and consent, more commonly without. If this is a problem in hospital-based psychiatry it is <u>a fortiori</u> a major issue in community psychiatry.

There are several practical issues which need attention. BASW has made a useful recommendation to social workers in its publication **Confidentiality in Social Work**, namely, that the social worker should seek to negotiate an explicit 'confidentiality contract' with the client, exploring explicitly with the client what information can be shared with colleagues and other agencies and which information is not to be divulged to others under any circumstances. Similarly the social worker should not make undertakings to receive confidences that he cannot keep and should make this clear to the client, or make clear in what circumstances and subject to what provisos he might be forced to divulge information if it was in the best interests of the client. These recommendations may well be applied to carers in other professions, or indeed to voluntary workers. Secondly, there is a question of how much information should be committed to writing in public records; clear policies should be developed as to what information is essential and what kinds of sensitive information it should be within the discretion of the professional to withhold. There are notorious difficulties about the protection of the confidentiality of medical records in public form in public institutions, and within a community setting these difficulties can be multiplied. Thirdly, there is a particular difficulty about the confidentiality of the 'extra' information gained when professionals and other helpers invade the privacy of the individual's home to interview and observe his family and friends at close quarters. Just as it is necessary to have rules and set limits to the extended confidentiality in the hospital team, so there is a pressing need to set limits to the number of people who have access to the privacy and confidences of vulnerable individuals and their families.

<u>The right to treatment</u>. The term 'treatment' is an ambiguous term in medicine generally and in psychiatry in particular. It covers both therapy and TLC (tender loving care). The right to treatment is normally interpreted as including the right to set limits to treatment and the right to refuse

treatment. There are clearly different modes in which professionals relate to patients depending on the severity of their disorder, and different degrees of freedom or responsibility to choose are allowed to the patient depending on the nature of his disorder and the stage of his recovery. The question arises whether patients treated at home or in the community have more or less freedom to choose the form and mode of their treatment. In theory the patient should have more independence on his own territory. In practice the situation may be very different.

The National Schizophrenia Fellowship has long campaigned for official recognition of the patient's right to follow-up after discharge from hospital, and the advocates of community psychiatry clearly support this view. However, this view of the NSF mainly represents the view of concerned relatives and may not represent the desires of discharged patients. Does a patient have a right to limit or terminate follow-up? A great deal depends on what is included in the follow-up package. Besides giving medication does it include supervising, rehabilitation, encouraging participation in self-help groups? Does it include a monitoring, surveillance remit or right of intervention to prevent the recurrence of a crisis? How far should lay volunteers/visitors and helpers be allowed to become involved? How many agencies becomes too much?

2. The Scope and Limits of Professional Duty
The duty to care is generally circumscribed by the declared or expressed need of the patient/client. At least in ordinary medicine the doctors right of intervention is limited to the self-defined problem of the person consulting him. Only in exceptional circumstances where the patient cannot be consulted or in an emergency can he act to deal with other problems not previously identified. This situation is more complicated but not essentially different where the patient is mentally disordered. Secondly, the right of follow-up or rehabilitation service is related to re-establishing the autonomy of the patient, not encouraging continuing dependency.

Against the background of these general principles a few brief comments on professional responsibilities will have to suffice. First, the duty to care means in this context that patients should not be forced into accepting hospitalisation if community care is available and would be better for them, or vice versa. Secondly, good team

management of patients in hospital or community
means that the participants need to have proper
training to develop the necessary skills to operate
effectively and efficiently in that mode. These are
not skills that are learnt by osmosis, and in
maintaining proper standards in the quality of care
given means not only willingness to undertake
appropriate in-service training, but a responsiblity
to educate professional colleagues. Similarly
working in the community in such a way as to promote
community involvement and self-help requires skills
which most health professionals do not automatically
possess, however well motivated they may be.

Thirdly, doctors, nurses and social workers
have to be aware of the ambiguous double role in
which they operate in psychiatry, whether in
hospital or community. This is most clearly illustrated in relation to supervising the 'dangerous' or
'criminally insane'. They are cast both in the role
of carers and ministers of therapy on the one hand
and agents of social control on the other. In the
first role there is a risk of paternalism and
dependency-creating modes of caring, in the second
role there is a risk of being seen in a quasi-
punitive or policing role. Properly understood, the
duty to care should help to correct the distortions
of these roles.

Fourthly, there needs to be much more clarity
about the sharing of responsiblity in the inter-
professional or multidisciplinary team. It is not
always clear who should lead the team, or who should
'carry the can'. The assumption of medical dominance
in leadership and decision-making may, in fact,
contradict the demands of proper rehabilitation.
Authority may be delegated but not abrogated by
doctors, and in some circumstances other
professionals should lead. However, training and
explicit negotiation about these matters should take
place if conflict is to be avoided or arbitrary
authority is not to defeat the ends of community
care and team co-operation.

Finally, the question must be asked whether
supervision by a community team encourages or dis-
courages the recovery of the patient and his ability
to assume responsibility for his own life. There are
risks of individuals and families in the community
becoming 'captive groups' and stigmatised in the
process by overweening professional involvement in
their lives and by being over-researched by
enthusiasts determined to prove a point about
community psychiatry.

3. Individual Needs, Community Involvement and
Responsibility
Justice demands that, in deciding how to deal with
individual needs, there should not only be objective
assessment of the best available means for dealing
with their needs, but also which means cause least
cost burden and inconvenience to families and the
rest of the community. As suggested earlier in this
chapter this means that there should be proper
assessment of costs and benefits, not just in cash
terms but in human terms. For example, is it fair to
impose on families the burden of care for mentally
disordered individuals, or to expect the community
to provide voluntarily support which might be part
of statutory services?
     Community-oriented services can only avoid
leading to deterioration of care for the mentally
disordered if attitudes are receptive to community
involvement. Current public attitudes to mental
illness and the stigma associated with it suggest
that a massive programme of education is necessary
before community psychiatry can really work. Has
adequate research been done on public attitudes and
how these can be changed? How do we educate the
media and the public to change stereotypical
attitudes to 'insanity'? How do we encourage the
public to take risks with previously identified
'dangerous' patients? Is there not a fear by lay
people and volunteers that they will be conscripted
into the role of agents of social control,
particularly if they become identified with official
community psychiatry initiatives, and lose the
access they have to people as voluntary counsellors
and advocates?
     How do we get people to respect the rights of
all men, including the elderly, the mentally
handicapped and the mentally disordered? This is a
major educational task and is perhaps the major
ethical issue in community psychiatry.

REFERENCE

Hawks D (1975). Community Care: An analysis of
    assumptions. British Journal of Psychiatry, 127,
    pp 276-285.

Chapter Five

STRAIGHTENING THE BEND: SOCIOLOGICAL CONTRIBUTIONS TOWARDS THE DEVELOPMENT OF COMMUNITY MENTAL HEALTH CARE

Geoffrey Baruch

Over the years there has been an uneasy relationship between sociologists and the medical profession, particularly psychiatrists. The criticism of the medical profession as imperialists seeking to take control of and dominate areas of social life is one that has also been levelled at sociologists (see Strong 1979). To put it crudely, our perception of medical activity has partly been motivated by our professional interest in establishing medical sociology as a legitimate area of study requiring a certain expertise. According to some sociologists, the advent of community psychiatry is a further instance of medicine unjustifiably involving itself in the problems of social life and treating deviant behaviour, formerly considered problematic in legal and moral terms, as a symptom of illness (see Scull 1977). The irony is that sociology contributed to this state of affairs. Having encouraged psychiatry to abandon the mental hospital and go out into the community, psychiatrists are once again charged with being imperialists.

I shall return to this issue towards the end of the paper when I briefly examine the work of Scott (1973) and Basaglia (1981). To begin with, I want to examine the contribution sociology made towards the development of community mental health care. Before doing so, I should say that the view I present is a personal and partial one and, certainly, open to question. Second, I shall not be assessing the importance of particular contributions nor shall I be suggesting that sociology was the only influence. Clearly, many factors have contributed to the development of community psychiatry including important clinical changes. Third, I am largely interested in ideas rather than practicalities although I shall consider some practical

implications.
    The theme which runs through most of the work I
shall   consider   is   the   view   of   medicine   and
psychiatry   as   an agent of social control. To argue
that medicine is engaged in 'social control' is   not
to   say doctors behave as a secret police force. All
it   means   is   that   medicine,   like   many   other
apparently   innocuous social activities like raising
children,   schooling   and   watching   television,
controls   aspects   of   knowledge   and   ideas   which
support the existing social   order   or   system   (see
Armstrong   1980).   To   give you an example, there is
unlikely to be dissent from the view of   members   of
society   and   a patient suffering from smallpox that
he should be quarantined although such   action   will
deprive   him   of   certain   rights and freedoms which
were previously taken   for   granted.   On   the   other
hand,   according   to   a minority of sociologists and
psychiatrists using ideas   derived   from   sociology,
such   issues   are   not   so   easily   resolved   in
psychiatry.   As   we   shall   see,   they   argued   that
psychiatry   rarely   promoted   health   but rather was
engaged almost exclusively in   controlling   deviance
and   maintaining   public   order.   Some   psychiatrists
agreed with the view; others, probably the majority,
disagreed   with   it,   but there is little doubt that
the   debate   about   social   control   has   been   an
important   influence   in   the   move away from mental
hospital care. Let us now consider some of the areas
in which this view has been advanced.

DEFINITIONS OF MENTAL ILLNESS

During   the   1950s   and   1960s   a   minority   of
psychiatrists and social scientists advanced the now
familiar   view that the disorders that psychiatrists
have come to regard as their proper concern are   not
medical problems at all (Morgan 1975). For instance,
Szasz (1961) argued that the idea of mental   illness
is   merely   a   'myth'   based   upon   the confused and
mistaken belief that bodily illness and   behavioural
disorders   should   be   explained   and treated alike.
According to Szasz, what psychiatrists call   mental
illness are problems of living, inextricably tied to
social and legal contexts that cannot   be   explained
in medical terms. He concludes that so-called mental
illness   should   be   removed   from   the   category   of
illnesses   and that it be regarded as the expression
of man's struggle with the problem of how he   should
live.   Similar   arguments   were   advanced   by Liefer
(1969). He claimed that while in medicine   'disease'

refers to phenomena that are not regulated by social custom, morality and law, but to undesired bodily structure and function, in psychiatry disease refers to behaviour which is subject to such regulation.

Others, like Wooton (1959) and Dunham (1967), took a less extreme view than Szasz and Liefer in not rejecting outright the relevance of the concept of mental illness to all psychological disorders but criticised its application to an unlimited diversity of social problems. A classic example was the crude application by some members of the social work profession of psycho-analytic notions to the problems presented by clients. Here clients' claims concerning material difficulties were interpreted as defences against psychological and emotional problems.

A third group of critics can be identified as the anti-psychiatrists who rejected the methodological assumptions and positivist practices of orthodox psychiatry. Their concern was with showing how schizophrenia was an existential problem and was therefore intelligible in these terms. Laing examined these issues first from a psychological/internal perspective in **The Divided Self** (1959) then in terms of family dynamics in **Sanity, Madness and the Family** (Laing & Esterson 1964) and finally in societal terms in **The Politics of Experience** (1967). At each stage, he broadened his concept of normality to the point where he argued that the schizophrenic's response was normal and rational and a valid political protest to the contradictions of capitalist society, whereas so-called normal members of society were those who were out of touch with reality. Laing's controversial views led to the introduction of settings in the community, like Kingsley Hall, whose equally controversial philosophy was consistent with the dangerous idea that the sufferer should be helped to regress so that he could be gradually reborn into sanity (see Barnes & Berke 1973).

Although all these views were unacceptable to the majority of psychiatrists, they stimulated a debate about the nature of psychiatric theory and practice both within the profession and in sections of the community (see Boyers & Orrill 1972, Friedenburg 1973). Leaving aside psychiatric objections, from a sociological perspective it can be argued that they explain away rather than explain the role of psychiatric definitions in society. The arguments I shall draw on have been most clearly presented in David Morgan's excellent paper

Explaining Mental Illness (1975). First, their views
are based on a misunderstanding of the relationship
between bodily and mental illness. All judgements
about what counts as illness as opposed to the
biological concept of disease have a social
component although this is rarely an issue much of
the time. Mechanic (1968) has illustrated this claim
in a most striking way in describing how 'dyschromic
spirochetosis, a disease characterised by spots of
various colours that appear on the skin, was so
common in a particular South American tribe that
Indians who did not have them were regarded as
abnormal and were even excluded from marriage' (p
16). Second, there is an important connection
between the way lay people and psychiatrists define
mental illness which is concerned with the way responsibility and intelligibility is not attributed to
certain types of deviant behaviour. Typically, an
action will be seen as indicating mental illness
from a lay point of view when it cannot be explained
in common sense terms. For instance, we immediately
understand why a woman who is divorced, has two
children and lives off social security shop-lifts,
whereas we would be hard put to take the same view
of a millionairess committing the same action. In
this case, we are likely to assume she is mentally
disturbed and not responsible for her behaviour.
Definitions in psychiatry, based as they are on
natural scientific criteria, are equally non-moral
in the way they do not attribute blame or responsibility in diagnosing mental illness. Morgan
(1975) has argued that regardless of its validity
psychiatric thought, like other modes of scientific
thought in our society, may provide a way of
neutralising the threat which unexplained, ir-
rational deviant behaviour poses to social order.
(In presenting this analysis, I have not done
justice to the richness and complexity of Morgan's
arguments nor have I mentioned the work of other
social scientists who, starting with the ideas of
the anti-psychiatrists, have contributed much to our
understanding of the meaning of mental illness (see
Ingleby 1981, 1982; Coulter 1973).)
    However, having made this criticism, there is
nevertheless little doubt that despite the ex-
travagant and excessive way in which the critics
made their claims, they promoted a climate which
made mental illness more understandable and less
threatening to non-sufferers. This provided a
further impetus to the already existing move towards
community forms of care.

THE MENTAL HOSPITAL

Equally, if not more important during the 1950s and
1960s, was the study of the psychiatric hospital as
a social institution. A number of studies sought to
show how psychiatric patients were dehumanised by
being denied freedom of will and were treated as
objects of technical and social control. Thus
hospitalisation did not promote health but prolonged
the chronic cause of the illness itself.

Let us briefly consider an example from Stanton
& Schwartz's classic study **The Mental Hospital**
(1954), which shows how institutional arrangements
and structure can adversely affect a patient's
behaviour. A catatonic patient's behaviour
deteriorated to a remarkable degree although
initially there appeared to the staff to be little
reason why this should be so. She spoke in such a
rapid manner that it was impossible to understand
her. Eventually the administrator of the hospital, a
psychiatrist, understood the word clothes in the
jumble of words and sentences coming from her. Her
clothes had been removed - as was the case for all
patients. Before the removal she had torn them, and
the superintendent had been advised by the patient's
psychotherapist not to let her have them or see
them. Thus they were stashed away in a locker and
this is what had led to the apparent deterioration
in her clinical presentation. The arrangements,
structure and processes of the institution had
contributed to this deterioration - the fact that it
was policy not to allow patients to wear clothes;
that the psychotherapist could tell the
superintendent what to do since his status was
higher. The patient's anxiety and odd behaviour were
resolved when the administrator told the patient
what had happened to her clothes and instructed the
superintendent to let her see them. Again,
institutional arrangements and structure made such a
resolution possible; for instance, the status of the
administrator was such that he could instruct the
superintendent.

Many studies appeared documenting similar
phenomena. One of the most influential was Goffman's
work on total institutions (1968). It is important
to understand that Goffman's analysis is based on a
theory of the self which, following the work of Mead
(see Morris 1967), argues that the self is socially
constructed in interaction with others. Thus total
institutions, like mental hospitals, develop
practices which are designed to strip away the

elements which previously constituted the inmates'
social identity and replace them with those relevant
to the easy maintenance of order in the institution.
For instance, laundering is a much simpler affair if
inmates wear regulation clothing rather than their
personal clothes. Moreover, regulation clothing
confirms the status of the wearer as a patient or
prisoner, whereas this might be open to question if
he was allowed to wear personal items of clothing.

Goffman's account of institutional life shows
how staff and patients have fundamentally different
points of view and may be hostile towards each
other. Advancement from back wards to discharge
wards may depend on conformist behaviour on the part
of the patient and not on improvements in his mental
health; decisions about discharge are made by
authority figures in the institution and the patient
has little or no say in the process; he has little
contact with the outside world and his daily round
of behaviour is heavily prescribed and takes place
almost exclusively within the confines of the
institution; the inmate has lost his previous social
roles such as parent, husband, employee and the only
way he can develop a non-institutional sense of self
is in secretive activities like finding used
cigarettes in hospital corridors and smoking them.
This is a deadening situation and leads to the loss
of social functioning that we usually take for
granted. A more balanced view of the institutional
life was presented by Wing & Brown (1970) in
Institutionalism and Schizophrenia but they
confirmed the negative effect on long-term patients
of a limited, institutionalised environment.

Like revelations about the institutional
treatment of the mentally handicapped, such studies
produced a sense of moral outrage which was not
altogether justified when one takes into account the
character of the mental hospital from an
organisational perspective. Following a model
developed by Perrow (1975), I think it is useful to
understand what happens to patients in a mental
hospital or any organisation for the care of
psychiatric patients in terms of three interacting
elements: structure, goals and technology. Structure
refers to the organisation of staff and patients so
that existing techniques can be carried out in order
to allow the achievement of goals. Technology refers
to the techniques available for reaching goals.
Goals are the objectives of the institution. This
model makes intelligible much of what I have
described about institutional life. Many of the

studies of mental hospitals were carried out at a
time when the new innovations in treatment,
particularly drug therapy, either had not made an
appearance or were just beginning to make an impact
so that the goals of hospitals cannot be said to
have been cure rather than control. The
unavailability of techniques also explains why those
best equipped to treat patients, the medical staff,
had the least contact with them and concentrated on
administrative duties. Crudely speaking, once the
new therapies were perceived as making an impact,
goals and structure changed, allowing for the
introduction of district general hospital psychiatry
and other forms of service within the community.

In summary, the many studies of the mental
hospital produced a climate which favoured their
abandonment.

THE PSYCHIATRIC PROFESSION

I shall be brief here, preferring to concentrate on
sociological research into the way people experience
mental illness and the implications of this work for
community psychiatry. From the perspective of the
sociology of the professions, it is important to
note that the move towards comprehensive district
based services with the district general hospital
psychiatric unit as the cornerstone of these
services has implications for the status of the
psychiatric profession. To put it simply, the
desegregation of the mentally ill involves the
desegregation of the profession and so brings it
into the mainstream of medicine. If you wish to
examine the development of the psychiatric
profession I recommend Scull (1979), Baruch &
Treacher (1978) and Jones (1972).

LAY METHODS OF RESPONDING TO PSYCHIATRIC ILLNESS

Critics of psychiatry have tended to ignore the role
of the patient and his 'significant others', usually
close relatives, in the process of social control.
According to them, the patient is unwilling to be
hospitalised but is coerced by the psychiatrists
into being admitted. This view has been challenged
by a minority of psychiatrists and sociologists,
using sociological ideas. Scott (1973, 1967, 1965)
and Bott (1976), following theories of the sick role
and illness behaviour developed by Mechanic (1962),
Parsons (1951) and Pilowsky (1969), have provided
important insights into the process of becoming

mentally ill and seeking hospitalisation. Their
ideas are also based on many years of experience as
a psychiatrist and psychotherapist at Napsbury
Hospital. Illness and the process of hospitalisation
start within family settings which Scott has had the
opportunity to study. His observations suggest that
many patients are able to use their madness not only
to influence and control their close relatives but
also to manipulate psychiatrists, social workers and
other professionals they encounter. Thus Scott's
work provides a different picture of the
psychiatrist/patient relationship from, for instance
the one presented by the anti-psychiatrists.
Certainly, the psychiatrist has great power in this
relationship but the patient is often in a position
to exploit the situation to his own advantage. For
instance, hospitalisation may be viewed by some
patients (and their close relatives) as a means of
avoiding difficult marital and family situations.
Moreover, this ability to exploit the 'sick role'
can turn into an inability ever to leave the role.
Any new therapeutic initiative taken by the
psychiatrist or other members of staff is dislocated
and eventually neutralised because neither the
patient nor his family can tolerate any fundamental
change.

Scott's concept, 'the treatment barrier',
describes the obstacles to effective treatment which
are created by the culturally prescribed view of
mental illness prevailing in Western society. As we
have seen, a central feature of this view is that
the mentally disordered are ill and hence lack
responsibility for their actions. According to Scott
and Bott, the mental hospital and what it represents
to the community is crucial in creating this
barrier. From my own research (Baruch & Treacher
1978), I have also come to the conclusion that the
mental hospital is an important factor in how
relatives perceive mental illness and its treatment.
However, I do not agree with an implication of
Scott's work that relatives, with the acquiesence of
the prospective patient, brazenly dispose of the
latter into the hospital setting. A number of
studies show that relatives play a vital role in the
hospitalisation process, but display a reluctance in
seeing psychiatric illness in the prospective
patient and in persuading him to seek help. The
research of Radke-Yarrow and her colleagues (1955)
found that wives of mentally ill husbands constantly
extended the barriers of normal behaviour in a
number of ways in order to interpret their

increasingly bizarre conduct within this framework
until this became impossible. However, I disagree
with the authors' explanation that such inter-
pretative activity occurs because relatives psychologically deny the reality of the illness due to its
threatening nature.

My own research has shown that relatives'
accounts of their involvement in the hospitalisation
process are constructed so as to appear moral. But
why should they have to justify the morality of
their actions? After all, encouraging someone who is
ill to seek treatment is usually considered as
appropriate conduct. However, the cultural meanings
attached to mental illness have a long history of
being associated with stigmatisation which is
evident in relatives' accounts. For instance,
although my research was about patients' and
relatives' experience of district general hospital
psychiatry, it was the local mental hospital which
figured prominently in their accounts as a
frightening place. (This may explain some of Agnes
Miles' findings in Chapter 6.) Thus relatives'
descriptions of how they constantly interpret and
re-interpret the patient's increasingly bizarre
behaviour in normal terms is a way of allowing for
the possibility that if they reported having taken
the first sign of such behaviour as indicating
psychiatric disturbance and advised hospitalisation
then their moral status would be open to question.
It is also striking how the relative consistently
appeals to the way he sought advice from a respected
outsider, like a local priest or a member of the
extended family who is close to the patient, as a
way of legitimising this decision before making an
appointment with the psychiatric services.

Other ways in which relatives establish their
good character include relating stories which
describe how they willingly put up and fall in with
the demands of the prospective patient even though
they appear unreasonable from the common sense
version of normality. For instance, the husband of a
patient described how he painstakingly deferred to
his wife's complaint that the kitchen floor was
dirty by removing the cooker from against the wall
on numerous occasions so that she could examine an
area of floor which had been hidden from view. In
making such descriptions, the husband is not only
providing evidence of his good character, but is
also demonstrating that his wife has an unsound
state of mind. After all, 'normal' people do not
need to judge the state of a kitchen floor by

looking behind the cooker on more than one occasion.
     It is at this stage that Scott's observations
are so important. Once the hospital confirms that
the patient is ill and requires admission, then the
relative believes that his view of the patient's
social behaviour as indicating an unsound state of
mind is legitimate and that he has no role to play
in the patient's problems or welfare. A fundamental
shift in identity has occurred; the patient's past
is open to re-interpretation and his future identity
may also be re-interpreted since health
professionals sanction illness. Finally, the
protracted nature of this process is liable to
weaken the effectiveness of therapeutic inter-
ventions.

CONCLUSIONS

Given this and other obstacles I have described,
community mental health care represents an advance
on treatment in mental hospital settings. However,
as I said at the beginning of the chapter, there are
some sociologists who do not see the change in
policy in this way. They argue that such a move
unjustifiably increases psychiatry's involvement in
the problems of social life. I think this claim is
based on the fundamental misconception that
regardless of the view one takes about the status of
'mental illness' people do not suffer in a way which
is massively real to them. Moreover it ignores the
potential for therapeutic innovations and change
which a community-based psychiatric service can
provide, particularly in overcoming the more
pernicious aspects of social control which I have
described. For instance, the work of Scott at
Napsbury and Barnet District General Hospital and
Basaglia in Trieste, Italy, is a response to the way
the mental hospital as an institution for
controlling deviance and maintaining public order
compromises psychiatry's goal for promoting health.
In both cases, the move towards treatment in the
community was a gradual one which initially involved
reforming the work of the mental hospitals from
which they operated and subsequently moving out into
the community (see Scott 1976, Basaglia 1981 for
detailed accounts of their practices). Although
their innovations may be little different from those
developed by other psychiatrists, I mention them
because they are based on the type of critique I
have developed in this chapter.
     Patients were said to go 'round the bend'

because many mental hospitals were built so that
they were hidden from the community by a bend in the
road. In straightening that bend, it is vital that
we do not entertain the idea that old practices
magically disappear. As Sansom-Fisher et al (1979)
show, staff can be as isolated from patients in a
general hospital psychiatric unit, as they appeared
to be in the studies on mental hospitals.

REFERENCES

Armstrong D (1980). An Outline of Sociology as
    Applied to Medicine. John Wright, Bristol.
Baruch G & Treacher A (1978). Psychiatry Observed.
    Routledge & Kegan Paul, London.
Basaglia F (1981). Breaking the Circuit of Control.
    Penguin, Harmondsworth.
Berke J & Barnes M (1973). Mary Barnes. Penguin,
    Harmondsworth.
Bott E (1976). Hospital and Society. British Journal
    of Medical Psychology, 49, pp 97-140.
Boyers R & Orril R (eds) (1972). Laing and Anti-
    Psychiatry. Penguin, Harmondsworth.
Coulter J (1973). Approaches to Insanity. Martin
    Robertson, London.
Dunham H W (1967). Community Psychiatry; the Newest
    Therapeutic Bandwagon. Current Issues in
    Psychiatry, 1, pp 289-302.
Friedenburg E Z (1973). Laing. Fontana, London.
Goffman E (1968). Asylums. Penguin, Harmondsworth.
Ingleby D (1981). Critical Psychiatry. Penguin,
    Harmondsworth.
Ingleby D (1982). The Social Construction of Mental
    Illness, in Wright P & Treacher A The Problem of
    Medical Knowlege. Edinburgh University Press.
Jones K (1972). A History of the Mental Health
    Service. Routledge & Kegan Paul, London.
Laing R (1959). The Divided Self. Tavistock, London.
Laing R & Esterson A (1964). Sanity, Madness and the
    Family. Tavistock, London.
Laing R (1967). The Politics of Experience. Penguin,
    Harmondsworth.
Liefer R (1969). In the Name of Mental Health.
    Science House, New York.
Mechanic D (1962). Some Factors in Identifying and
    Defining Mental Illness. Mental Hygiene, 46, 66-74

Mechanic D (1968). _Medical Sociology_. The Free
    Press, New York.
Morgan D (1975). Explaining Mental Illness. _Archives
    of European Sociology_, 16, pp 262-280.
Morris C W (ed) (1967). _Mind, Self and Society_.
    Phoenix Edition, University of Chicago Press,
    Chicago.
Parsons T (1951). _The Social System_. Free Press,
    Chicago.
Perrow C (1975). Hospitals, Technology, Structure
    and Goals, reprinted in March J G (ed) _Handbook of
    Organisations_. Rand McNally, Chicago.
Pilowsky I (1969). Abnormal Illness Behaviour.
    British Journal of Medical Psychology, 42, 347-351
Radke-Yarrow M, Schwartz C G, Murphy H S & Deary L C
    (1955). The Psychological Meaning of Mental
    Illness in the Family. _Journal of Social Issues_,
    11, pp 12-24.
Sansom-Fisher R W, Desmond Poole A & Thomson V
    (1979). Behaviour Patterns within a General
    Hospital Psychiatric Unit: An Observational Study.
    Behaviour Research and Therapy, 17, pp 317-332.
Scott R D & Ashworth P L (1965). The 'Axis Value'
    and the Transfer of Psychosis; a Scored Analysis
    of the Interaction in the Families of
    Schizophrenic Patients. _British Journal of Medical
    Psychology_, 38, pp 97-116.
Scott R D & Ashworth P L (1967). 'Closure' at the
    First Schizophrenic Breakdown: a Family Study.
    British Journal of Medical Psychology, 40, pp 109-
    145.
Scott R D (1973). The Treatment Barrier, Part 1.
    British Journal of Medical Psychology, 46, pp 45-
    55.
Scull A C (1979). _Museums of Madness_. Allen Lane,
    London.
Scull A C (1977). _Decarceration_. Prentice Hall,
    Englewood Cliffs, New Jersey.
Stanton A H & Schwartz M S (1954). _The Mental
    Hospital_. Basic Books, New York.
Strong P (1979). Sociological Imperialism and the
    Profession of Medicine: a Critical Examination of
    the Thesis of Medical Imperialism. _Social Science
    and Medicine_, 13a, pp 199-215.
Szasz T (1961). _The Myth of Mental Illness_. Harper
    Row, Newcastle.
Wing J & Brown G W (1970). _Institutionalism and
    Schizophrenia_. Cambridge University Press,
    Cambridge.
Wooton B (1959). _Social Science and Social
    Pathology_. Allen & Unwin, London.

Chapter Six

THE STIGMA OF PSYCHIATRIC DISORDER: A SOCIOLOGICAL PERSPECTIVE AND RESEARCH REPORT

Agnes Miles

It is commonly observed that mental illness carries a stigma. Professionals and lay people alike refer to the 'stigma of mental illness' as though it were an accepted item of general knowledge. But for sociologists, stigma is an elusive and difficult concept which medical sociologists have been struggling for a long time to clarify, especially in relation to mental illness.

In sociological literature Goffman's influential discussion on stigma (Goffman 1963) is often taken as a starting point. Following Goffman, stigma can be defined as an attribute, characteristic or condition which is evaluated by society as undesirable. This is a very broad definition, as one can argue that all types of illness, physical as well as mental, are stigmatised in this sense, ill health in general being evaluated as something bad and undesirable. However, there are a number of sociological features, common to all stigmatised states, the consideration of which helps to clarify the meaning of stigma:

1. The stigmatised attribute is seen as so important, so distinguishing, that the person possessing it becomes defined in terms of that one attribute. Thus, someone may come to be defined by his social group as the 'cripple', the 'blind man', the 'simpleton' or the 'madman', the whole person, therefore, becoming stigmatised.
2. The stigmatised one is devalued, seen by the social group as less acceptable, and less desirable than others. Stigma is discrediting and in Goffman's words a person's identity becomes 'spoiled'.
3. Inherent in the notion of stigma is some

measure of permanency, of its being difficult
to shake off, lasting if not necessarily all
the rest of one's life, at least for some
considerable time.

Thus, when we say that mental illness carries a
stigma, we mean that it is so negatively evaluated
by society, so much seen as undesirable and
discrediting, as to result in marking, more or less
permanently, the whole person who has been identified as mentally ill.
From a sociological point of view there are a
number of controversial issues surrounding the
stigma attached to mental illness. I want to mention
briefly a few such issues, namely those to which my
current research may make some contribution.
At what stage does a person become identified
as mentally ill by the social group? When is stigma
attached? Researchers during the 1950s and 1960s
showed that admission to a mental hospital was the
turning point. According to Cumming, 'mental
illness, it seems, is a condition which afflicts
people who go to a mental institution, but up until
they go, almost anything they do is fairly normal'
(Cumming & Cumming 1957: 102). Admission is the
specific event which brings about changes of status.
However, with changes in the treatment and
management of psychiatric illness, there are now
many patients who receive treatment on an outpatient
basis. The question arises, therefore, as to whether
stigma is attached to being a psychiatric patient if
this does not involve hospitalisation. Moreover,
many of those who are admitted enter the psychiatric
units of general hospitals; is being a patient in
such a unit less stigmatising?
If the Cummings and other early researchers are
right, it would seem that it is not so much the
disturbed behaviour but the hospital admission which
brings about stigma. Clearly, there must be some
exceptions; behaviour which seems very bizarre to
the social group may well mark a person as 'mad' in
or out of hospital; but it is possible that some
depressed, withdrawn patients would not be
stigmatised without the event of admission.
These issues lead to another: how lasting is
the stigma of mental illness? According to some
sociologists stigma is very lasting; they argue that
admission to a mental hospital constitutes public
labelling and that after discharge a patient becomes
known as an 'ex-patient' much as a discharged
prisoner becomes known as an 'ex-prisoner', a role

very difficult to reverse. (For a review of the literature, see Miles 1981.) Other researchers have argued, however, that the opposite can also happen, that after a time stigma disappears and that where the stigmatising 'ex-patient' role continues, this is due to the continued disturbed behaviour, or to relapses, rather than to the fact of once having been in a mental hospital (Gove 1970, Kirk 1974).

These points are not mere sociological niceties for academic argument, but have practical implications for the rehabilitation and management of the mentally ill. For example, if mental hospital stay is so stigmatising that an individual's future standing in his social group, and prospects of employment are damaged by it, then perhaps admission should be avoided, if at all possible. If psychiatric outpatient treatment can also damage a person's future chances, then treatment given in the surgeries of general practitioners may be preferable.

There are many important questions but little reliable information. The issues are important because the consequence of stigma can be devastating - social relationships, self esteem, employment chances, and the respect of one's fellows, can all be affected.

The paucity of research on the stigma of mental illness is due, at least partially, to the serious problems caused by designing and carrying out empirical research in this field. It is extremely difficult to operationalise the concept of stigma, and to separate the various elements inherent in the situation of someone who is stigmatised. For example, a feeling that one is actually experiencing stigmatisation by others is an element which has to be distinguished from that person's anxiety and expectation that such stigmatisation would occur; and feelings and expectations of stigma have to be distinguished from actual social processes occurring within the social group.

When patients and ex-patients struggle with their anxieties and try to make sense of their experiences of stigma they are seldom lucid, and researchers have tremendous difficulties in interpreting what such patients say. I would like to illustrate this by quoting two remarks from my current research: one patient said 'I do not feel that I have a stigma, I just feel rejected by everybody'; and another said 'I do not feel stigmatised, I just think that everybody says I should be'.

I turn now to my present research which is concerned with the social networks of psychiatric patients and with the social support given to such patients, in Southampton. The study of stigma is a relatively small, though important, aspect of this study. The research is ongoing, and I can give only some preliminary findings.

The sample consists of patients diagnosed by psychiatrists as suffering from a neurotic disorder. Both men and women are included in the sample: all are married, living with their spouses, and are of working age. They all received treatment on an outpatient basis and none had inpatient treatment at any time. In fact, most are first referrals.

Rather lengthy interviews are being conducted with patients in their homes; so far 75 patients have been interviewed. An interview schedule designed by the MRC Psychiatry Unit in Australia (Interview Schedule for Social Interaction) is being used. After an interval of one year, patients will be re-interviewed in order to see whether changes in their relationships and circumstances have occurred. The interview material reveals the patients' reported feelings and experiences concerning stigma; no 'objective' measure of their feelings and experiences is available. I will now mention briefly some findings.

1. Many patients felt stigmatised; they either talked of rejection by their former networks (friends, relatives, neighbours), or of being treated differently (in a negative sense) by them, compared with the pre-illness situation. Patients said that former friends or colleagues turned away from them: 'They think I am funny', 'They avoid me', 'They do not come around any more'. One man said, 'I have sudden panics, I used to think it was a heart attack, but now I know it is nerves. My boss is very good, he gave me a different job, but he said "don't tell the others, they will be at me to give you the sack, if they they think you are a loony, you know". I felt terrible when he said that'. Both men and women expressed this feeling of being rejected and stigmatised.

2. As mentioned before, all of the patients in the research are outpatients; they attend sessions at the psychiatric unit of a large general hospital. This unit is housed in a large modern block, and was opened only four or five years ago; it is a nice building, and freshly

painted. Nevertheless, many patients feel attendence to be stigmatising. According to one woman: 'I was waiting for my appointment in the lobby when a couple sat down next to me. The man said "I suppose you are waiting for visiting time like us"; I did not say anything, so he went on: "I don't like visiting here, they are loonies after all, and the worst is they look the same as us, so you don't know how bad they are, I reckon they should shut them away more". When he said this, I felt terrible - I felt so humiliated'. From this study I cannot tell whether the situation may be worse at the local psychiatric hospital, which is an old hospital some way away from Southampton. But attending the new hospital unit is certainly not problem-free.

3. As none of these patients is an inpatient, nor ever has been, the stigma they talk about is clearly not the consequence of hospital admission. The feeling of stigma seems to be there following the sequence of psychiatric symptoms, referral to a psychiatrist and treatment. It is a package; and it is not possible to say whether it was the patient's symptoms that brought about the feeling of stigma, or the fact of referral to a psychiatrist and psychiatric treatment. The patients themselves feel that stigma is the consequence of going to a psychiatrist and attending a psychiatric unit, rather than the consequence of any problems or symptoms that they have.

4. Not only acquaintances, neighbours and workmates but also relatives and close, long-standing friends were reported as having rejected the patients. One woman said that her mother did not visit her any more and told everyone in the family not to do so either; another said her sister stopped inviting her for Christmas. They attributed rejection, by mother and sister, to psychiatric referral and treatment, respectively.

5. It may seem amazing, in these circumstances, that all patients reported that their having psychiatric treatment was known to their networks of friends, relatives, etc. Few tried concealment - they told people themselves or their spouses did.

6. It is interesting to note that patients, when referring to psychiatric illness, used

terminology such as 'loony', 'mental', 'nuts', 'crazy'. They attributed these words to others, and thought that people referred to them in such terms.

Of course, social expectations regarding stigma are strong. As Goffman said, when people acquire a stigmatised characteristic or condition such as mental illness in adult life, a peculiar situation can arise. Individuals who have known and shared the values of their social group have strong expectations as to how others will behave towards themselves in a given situation. A patient receiving psychiatric treatment for the first time would know how he himself had felt towards psychiatric patients, in the past.

In conclusion, I would say that feelings of stigma and rejection exist, attaching not only to admission to a mental illness hospital, and not only to treatment for long-term disabling psychiatric illness. It seems also to follow treatment for a neurotic disorder at an outpatient clinic of a general hospital. These are rather gloomy findings, but I would hesitate to argue from these preliminary results that the policy of putting more emphasis on outpatient treatment in psychiatric units of general hospitals will not help to reduce stigma in the long run. Rather, I would say that the problem is great; social expectations and social values go very deep and change more slowly than we sometimes hope.

As a final footnote, I would like to answer a question many people have asked me - 'why did you choose neurotics?' I have always worked with long-stay patients before, but since starting this research, I have become rather a 'champion' of neurotic patients. To continue the Cinderella analogy, neurotics seem to be the Cinderellas of the medical and psychiatric services, in that they experience deep, long-term suffering and are neglected by professionals and lay people alike. This is understandable in that neurotics lack what sociologists call 'social visibility' - they are less likely to produce crisis situations or become public nuisances than psychotics, so they can be neglected. They can also be extremely irritating; their very symptoms can be very irritating to professionals and lay people alike, and quite often both groups find it difficult to accept them as sick. I think that neurotics are not only very isolated, especially the women who do not work; they are very lonely and their suffering may continue for many years. They need rehabilitation as much as anybody else, but they are neglected and receive little help.

REFERENCES

Cumming E & Cumming J (1957). Closed Ranks. Harvard University Press, Cambridge, Mass.
Cumming J & Cumming E (1968). On the Stigma of Mental Illness, in Spitzer S P & Denzin N K (eds), The Mental Patient. McGraw-Hill, New York.
Goffman E (1963). Stigma. Prentice Hall, New York.
Gove W R (1970) Societal reaction on an explanation of mental illness: an evaluation. American Sociological Review, 35, pp 873.
Kirk S A (1974). The impact of labelling on rejection of the mentally ill. Journal of Health and Social Behaviour, 15, pp 108
Miles A (1981). The Mentally Ill in Contemporary Society. Martin Robertson, Oxford.

PART TWO

PLANNING THE IDEAL SERVICE: CLINICAL AND NON-CLINICAL ELEMENTS

The chapters in Part Two take us on from theoretical considerations to deal with the questions which arise at the stage of planning both new services and modifications and additions to existing ones. Two main papers were presented at the conference in order to cover the range of elements which could constitute an ideal service. Even so, both authors had to be selective in the topics they chose to include. Dr John Reed's chapter owes much to his experiences as a consultant psychiatrist in the forefront of many developments in the psychiatric service in the City and Hackney Health District following its divorce from its back-up mental illness hospital in 1974. His wholehearted advocacy of locally-based services is tempered somewhat in the discussion by Dr Bernard Heine, whose experience in a large mental illness hospital, linked to two district general hospitals units, leads him to reassert some of the better points of that pattern of care.

The second chapter in this section, by Adrian Lovett, likewise reflects its author's work in Hackney as a senior officer in the local authority's Comprehensive Housing Service. The chapter offers encouragement and ideas to many whose plans for progress are thwarted by lack of 'ordinary' accommodation for their patients. The case for special projects and housing association involvement is succinctly and persuasively put in Ian Diamant's discussion.

Subjects selected for more detailed discussion in chapters arising from the seminar sessions are problems in planning a local service; how the planning process works; the nursing element; the planning of a psychiatric intensive care unit; and ways of bridging the gap between hospital and home.

Chapter Seven

THE ELEMENTS OF AN IDEAL SERVICE: THE CLINICAL VIEW

John Reed

In discussing the clinician's view of the development of comprehensive locally-based psychiatric services, I would like to set my remarks in context by some consideration of the historical background to such services. It also gives me the opportunity to point out that this is not the first time in the history of British psychiatry that London University and St Bartholomew's Hospital have been in the forefront of developments of such services.

Of the many members of the Tuke family who were involved in the development of adequate and humane treatment for the mentally ill in the nineteenth century, Daniel Hack Tuke was a student at St Bartholomew's before becoming Superintendent of The Retreat at York, a hospital which largely managed to resist the tendency in the second half of the nineteenth century towards the development of large custodial institutions. John Connolly, the first Professor of Medicine in the University of London, was the first doctor to suggest that a mental health service should be based in a local hospital and should provide 'not only inpatient accommodation, but also a domiciliary service supervised by a rotating panel of doctors and nurses from its staff'. In this way he hoped it would be possible to treat in their own homes a large proportion of patients who would otherwise have to be admitted. As Professor of Medicine, he had some remarks to make on teaching and suggested that each lunatic asylum should become 'a clinical school in which medical students might prepare themselves for their future duties'. On a more fanciful level I can even draw your attention to an earlier psychiatrist called John Reid who was a physician to the Finsbury Dispensary in London at the beginning of the

nineteeenth century. He showed that, as well as
being helpful, institutional life could be harmful
and that asylums could become 'nurseries for and
manufactories of madness', rather than hospitals for
recovery and cure. So here in City and Hackney we
are following instructions left to us by others.

At the beginning of the nineteenth century a
number of small and very effective hospitals for the
mentally ill were founded as a reaction against the
appalling conditions under which the mentally ill
were living in the community and prisons. For
reasons that are not entirely clear, this movement
did not spread across the whole country and perhaps
as a reaction against over-optimism an attitude of
moral blame towards the mentally ill began to
replace the attitude of moral treatment. There was a
return towards a view which equated insanity and
crime and a movement towards similar solutions for
all people presenting socially unacceptable
behaviour. Criminals were transported to Botany Bay,
lunatics were transported to big mental
institutions, which were almost as isolated, though
not so many miles away. Management of all types of
social deviance was based on the expulsion from
society of the deviant person until such time that
'reformation through management and education could
take place'. These attitudes were reflected in the
Lunacy Acts of 1890 and 1891, and led to the
creation of huge institutions for the mentally ill
with large numbers of patients admitted to hospital
for very long periods of time.

The situation began to change again in the late
1920s and early 1930s. Again the reason for this is
not entirely clear to me though I suspect that it
may reflect the experiences of doctors and of the
public at large in the management of shell-shock
cases from the First World War and the success of
some doctors in their management. A new, more open,
attitude towards the management of mental illness
developed and was reflected in the Mental Treatment
Act, 1939.

The Second World War appears to have influenced
further changes in the development of psychiatric
care, with a move away from large institutions and
increased emphasis on the social element of
treatment. Following the war there was a
considerable influx of new doctors, again with
experience of management of acute psychiatric states
and of the problems of institutionalisation arising
from the rehabilitation of returning prisoners of
war. One psychiatrist, Max Glatt, has graphically

described the development of institutionalisation in
normal internees, himself included. Within certain
hospitals, such as Mapperley and Netherne, a new
regime of open wards, therapeutic communities and an
emphasis on rehabilitation rather than containment
became prominent. In these hospitals it was found
that, even before the introduction of psychotropic
drugs such as chlorpromazine in 1955, there was a
decreasing number of inpatients. These changes were
formalised in the passing of the Mental Health Act
in 1959. In 1962 the 'Hospital Plan' was published.
This proposed that psychiatric units attached to
district general hospitals would be able to meet the
needs of most acute psychiatry with longer-term
illness such as patients with severe dementia being
managed in local community hospitals. **Better
Services for the Mentally Ill** (DHSS 1975) among
other things, reviewed progress towards achieving
that end, and noted that non-hospital based
facilities remained minimal in most areas. The
failure to provide adequate services was said to be
'the greatest disappointment of the last 15 years'.
    In City and Hackney Health District we have
gone some way towards providing a truly comprehensive district service. We have here an inner-
urban catchment area of approximately 188,500
people. The district covers one of the most
seriously deprived inner-city areas in London,
rating extremely high on most indicators of social
deprivation. Yet since 1974 the psychiatric service
has been operating independently of any large
psychiatric hospital and provides wide-ranging
services for young and old patients with either
mental illness or mental handicap. The only patients
who have to be treated outside the district are
those needing conditions of security, attainable
only in the special hospitals and a very small
number (four on average) of patients who need semi-
secure accommodation. We will be able to provide for
this latter group ourselves within the next four
years.
    In planning this service, various factors which
were not previously apparent have become clearer. It
is more obvious now that all elements of the service
are of equal importance and are inextricably
interlinked. Deficiency in one area will put
additional strain on another; over-provision of one
element will not compensate for under-provision of
another. For instance if there are too few hospital
beds then there will be an intolerable pressure on
community care services and on the community itself.

On the other hand if there are too many beds then
they will inevitably be used, patients will stay in
hospital unnecessarily and problems of
institutionalisation will develop which will
increase the difficulties of the rehabilitation and
community services.

In discussing the various elements of a service
the following should be considered:

1. <u>Hospital beds</u>. Questions have been raised,
   notably in Italy, about the need for anything
   other than the minimum of hospital beds. It is
   clearly not practical, in terms of present
   knowledge, to dispense with beds entirely.
   However, the proportion of beds needed, and the
   relationships between bed needs, admissions
   policies and the provison of other treatment
   facilities is ill-understood, and the report of
   an investigation jointly between the Royal
   College of Psychiatrists and the Health
   Advisory Service to look at the relationships
   between bed needs and the provision of other
   facilities is eagerly awaited. The document
   from the DHSS on planning and bed norms which
   emphasises that there is no one correct norm is
   extremely important. The number of beds that a
   district may need can only be determined in the
   light of an overall operational policy for that
   district. At present we are working with
   roughly 0.6 beds per thousand population; I
   suspect that we will find as we develop our
   community services further and our services for
   the elderly that some hospital beds will become
   superfluous.

   Adequate provision (beds and full range of
   supporting services) for the elderly - not only
   the elderly mentally infirm but all elderly
   patients - is probably the most important
   aspect of providing effective local services.
   Unless elderly patients are adequately provided
   for, facilities for younger patients will
   inevitably be taken over by longer-term elderly
   patients. Perhaps the recent suggestion of an
   overall bed allocation, with a division between
   beds for elderly and younger patients agreed
   locally, shows a way forward.

2. <u>Outpatient clinics</u>. In a community-oriented
   service it is necessary to make greatly
   increased provision for outpatient clinics, not
   only for new and short-term patients, but to

accommodate the large proportions of chronically ill patients who are maintained outside hospital as part of the community care programme. We are now running approximately three times the number of psychiatric outpatient clinics suggested by DHSS norms and in addition we find an increasing need for clinics (run principally here by community psychiatric nurses with medical support and supervision) for patients on long-term psychotropic medication by injection.

3. Emergencies. Evidence both from hospitals running a crisis intervention team and from local experience of running an emergency clinic shows that an effective service for dealing with emergencies plays a large part in avoiding admission to hospital. What is not clear is what type of service is best for dealing with emergencies. What is most effective may well depend on the area being served. Crisis intervention has been extensively written up, is well established and has proven its worth. Hospital-based emergency clinics, such as the one at Hackney Hospital and the one run by the Maudsley Hospital, are also effective. An emergency clinic might not reach all those helped by a crisis intervention service, but it is somewhat more economic to run and probably better at dealing with short-term problems. A third possibility for emergencies is a community mental health centre such as at Handen Road in Lewisham or Brindle House in Hyde. It is not entirely clear how far this type of emergency service deals with mentally ill people who, under other arrangements, come to the notice of psychiatrists, and how far it attracts part of the wider range of people showing 'conspicuous psychiatric morbidity' described by Goldberg (Goldberg & Huxley 1980).

4. Day hospitals and rehabilitation. Separate day hospital services for elderly and younger patients are necessary. Ideally these day hospitals should be organised separately from the occupational therapy facilities for inpatients. The shorter-term aims of inpatient occupational therapy frequently conflict with the longer-term aims and programmes of day hospital treatment. In addition to more traditional occupational therapy, emphasis must be

placed on learning social skills and on
handling social relationships. Conventional
attitudes towards rehabilitation have tended to
emphasise the needs for occupational rehabilitation, and to have been 'prescribed' as
a course of treatment over a defined period of
time, after which the patient may be considered
to have 'failed' if the outcome is not
immediately successful. This should no longer
be true either for 'old' long-stay or for
younger chronically mentally ill patients. For
this latter group it is important to ensure
that the patient has the opportunity to settle
in satisfactory accommodation outside the
hospital, as a base for developing social and
working skills. Maslow's theory of the
hierarchy of needs (which may be summarised as
saying that it is not usually realistic to work
towards self-fulfilment through work, or higher
goals unless you are first able to satisfy
lower level needs, such as knowing where you
are going to lay your head that night, or get
your next meal) is a relevant, but often
ignored, factor in planning the pattern of
rehabilitation for chronically ill patients.

5. 'Old' long-stay patients. In the development of
comprehensive district-based services it could
be argued that it would be ideal for each
district to manage locally all the old long-
stay patients from the big psychiatric
hospitals. We have not attempted to take all
patients from other hospitals, but we take over
the medical care of all those who can be
discharged, and who still have active contacts
in this district. Two main factors prevent
patients returning to the district from which
they originated. Firstly, there are some
patients who are not well enough to be discharged. Secondly, there are other patients,
probably the larger number, who no longer have
any meaningful contact in their area of origin,
and who refuse to be returned on the basis of a
'settlement certificate' to a place they left
perhaps 40 years ago. This is an attitude with
which clinicians and planners should be
entirely in sympathy. One of the few major
problems that we have had with the 'old' long-
stay returning to Hackney centred on such a
difficulty. One ex-patient set fire to his
lodgings, not because he wanted to get back

into hospital, but because he wanted to be
transferred to live in Epsom, having lived
there, albeit in hospital, for 20 years, and
which he had come to regard as his home. With
the 'Care in the Community' provisions it may
be possible to look further at the needs of
people such as this, and see what facilities
can be offered to suit them.

Considerable evidence is being published (see,
for instance, Wing 1982, Bewley et al. 1981) that
there is a problem of accumulation of patients
needing long-term hospital care - the 'new' long-
stay. We have, in this district, large numbers of
chronically mentally ill patients. A survey of a
one-year patient cohort (Lomas 1979) showed 715
people who were categorised as having a chronic
illness, and who were in current contact with the
hospital psychiatric service. However, there were no
young (under 65) mentally ill people whom the
consultants considered in need of long-term hospital
inpatient care. Why is there this discrepancy?
Although the complete answer is not clear, some
possible contributing factors may be considered. One
obvious reason for our not having a 'long-stay'
category is that we do not have longer-stay beds
assigned in which to put patients. If someone is in
hospital here they are on an acute ward, and like
all our patients are reviewed every week. The
doctors, nurses and social workers live day-by-day,
week-by-week, month-by-month with their failures.
This is not a comfortable situation and leads to the
search for more satisfactory ways of managing the
chronically ill. The fact that we have few beds
serves to encourage us to reserve beds for the most
severely disturbed patients and to discharge
patients as soon as their health improves. It is
possible that a result of such a policy could be
that some patients, chronically ill, and in need of
asylum and a great deal of practical help, are in
the community and suffering from so-called
decarceration - in other words, living highly
deprived, unsupported lives at considerable cost to
themselves and to the community in general. This has
been shown many times to be the lot of patients
discharged to inadequate or absent community support
and care. It has not been shown to occur where
specialised community services are developed and
easily accessible. An insulin-dependent diabetic may
well become comatose and die if discharged from
hospital with inadequate information, no support

from doctors or a clinic and with only a limited
supply of insulin. We have not kept all insulin-
dependent diabetics in hospital but have created a
service suited to their needs in the localities in
which they live. Exactly the same principles should
be true for people who are chronically mentally ill
or disabled.

   This leads to another possible reason for the
different findings about the existence of 'new'
long-stay patients. During the initial survey we
acquired an assessment not only of patients' medical
state, but about appropriate accommodation and day-
time occupation. We found that a sizable proportion
of chronically ill patients were assessed to be
inappropriately housed, and inappropriately occupied. Inevitably the needs of the patients in
terms of accommodation and occupation were much more
varied than the facilities available, both in and
out of hospital. Clinicians and social workers were
constantly hammering 'round' patients into 'square'
hostels; not unnaturally the result was a very high
readmission rate. This was a problem that had to be
solved urgently and I must express my deepest thanks
on behalf of the mentally ill in Hackney, to the
Gatsby Charitable Foundation which has enabled us to
develop a variety of experimental projects, also to
the local housing and social services departments
for their invaluable support in the development of
sheltered accommodation and occupational projects
for the chronically ill. Our local District
Management Team also has been a great help in
encouraging innovation and exploration of
alternative styles of care. This district now has
conventional hostels and group homes, communal
homes, a flatshare scheme using council flats, a
specially supported block of ten flats,
volunteer/befriending scheme, Industrial Education
Unit and occupation liaison workers. With the
teamwork of an enormous number of people, some
already mentioned and many more besides, we have
gone some considerable way to provide an adequate
framework for community care.

   Bricks and mortar, however elegant and suited
to an individual's needs, are no substitute for a
proper social network - friends, acquaintances and
professional carers. We now have a well developed
community psychiatric nursing service with 16 nurses
and a nursing officer, specialised and experienced
hospital social workers and, to fill the gaps,
people working specifically in the field of helping
people to settle into satisfactory accommodation,

and, in due course, jobs or day-time occupation. The
most common reason for a chronically mentally ill
person to lose a job is not because of inability to
cope with the technical aspect of the work, but
because of the loss of (or non-acquisition of)
social skills necessary to function at work. The
main thrust of work now is on the social disabilities of mental illness.

What effects, therefore, do community
developments like these have on the hospital? In the
three years or so since we began to develop a more
effective service directed towards the chronically
mentally ill our readmissions have dropped while our
first admissions have increased slightly, with the
total number of admissions remaining constant around
900 each year. We interpret this to indicate that
inpatient beds and other facilities are now being
used more to treat acutely ill patients rather than
those who return to hospital with a substantial
social component to their psychiatric problem and
who do not need full hospital care. The chronically
mentally ill who might well have become 'new' long-
stay in other districts are now leading satisfying
lives (to judge from their own remarks) in the
community, in accommodation more suited to their
needs and capabilities than a hospital ward.

I believe that not only is it possible to
provide a virtually comprehensive district-based
psychiatric service, even though there can be no one
ideal model, but also that this is preferable to a
service with a remote hospital. I also think that a
local service must inevitably become, with the
hospital as part of the network, community-oriented.
I would urge planners, and my colleagues, to
recognise the necessity of concentrating at least as
much on the needs of the chronically ill as on those
of the more acutely ill. The chief advantage of a
local service from the clinician's point of view is
that one is inevitably made aware of unmet and
changing needs; likewise one is in a relatively good
position - and well motivated - to improve the
service and meet those needs.

DISCUSSION AND COMMENTS

Bernard Heine

Runwell Hospital, where I work, was built in the 1930s with 850 beds. It has links with two district general hospital (DGH) units. The large hospital, itself, is some distance from the community and so we live with the kind of problems that trouble similar large establishments. It is from this background that I wish to discuss the provision of clinical services for mental illness. Some 12 years ago the North East Thames Regional Health Authority confronted our hospital with the plan of closure. It was thought to be a lethal contact but, in fact, it produced such a concentration of minds that we are now bottom of the list for closure. However, two other large hospitals in this region, Friern Barnet and Claybury, have been earmarked for closure. This has again led to an analysis of current psychiatric services. It is, therefore, useful to consider what special services large psychiatric hospitals can offer and how to provide adequate or better alternatives.

It is unfortunate to associate automatically the term 'institution' with being 'bad'. A prison is usually seen as a bad institution with its rigid hierarchy, its inmates at the lowest level, and loss of individuality. One can see how some of those characteristics developed in the large hospitals and how the condition of institutionalisation developed. Changes have occurred, and I agree with John Reed that these began even before the introduction of tranquillisers. One should note that the catalyst was often powerful, if benevolent, medical superintendents.

More recently, bed numbers have decreased, staffing ratios have increased and the image of the large psychiatric hospital has improved. Further stimuli for this came from pressure groups such as Community Health Councils, MIND and the Hospital Advisory Service. However, because of the sheer size of a large hospital, there can be inertia and a feeling of stasis. One overriding problem can be the distance from the local community. So, whilst one is not maintaining that a large institution should remain in its present form, it is pertinent to look at the services it provides, and to ensure that district community services can provide alternatives that are adequate and of similar quality, or better.

One alternative is to have not a large hospital for each district but what is termed a 'zone' hospital, providing a supra-district service. It may be seen as a resource centre. A key resource to be provided is for those small groups of patients in each district which pose problems of care. They are small in number, difficult to treat and need specialised units. Examples are: mentally ill offenders, disturbed adolescents, the older age group of constantly disturbed personalities and, of course, the 'new' chronic sick. Some disturbed adolescents and mentally ill offenders are having to be cared for in large, private hospitals; a reflection on our National Health Service.

Psychiatric services in City and Hackney are distinctive. The unit is in London; there is a large academic input and there is an excellent range of very stimulating staff. This does not always occur in isolated, small DGH units and a broad range of treatment settings is difficult to provide in such a unit. As to staff, a larger resource centre would be able to employ larger numbers of staff, offer possibilities of specialised training and provide a focus for research. But to overcome any sense of isolation, I believe that staff who work in resource centres should also have links with DGH units. So one is not thinking of alternatives but of resource centres providing specialised services as part of an integrated system.

To return to DGH units; I believe they have limitations. Part of my work is in a DGH unit and it always interests me to see the number of what I would call 'sophisticated patients' who prefer to go to the larger hospital, despite its greater stigma. They find it more caring and comfortable, with less emphasis on a highly-organised programme geared to early discharge. In DGH units this can be of overriding concern but as far as I can see, patients do not stay very much longer in the more comfortable large hospital, nor do they suffer therapeutically. It seems regrettable, to me, that hospital admission for psychiatric patients is so often seen as a last resort and I do not much care for statistics which show that community services reduce hospital admissions. To my mind it is quite appropriate, in a crisis, to admit patients perhaps for largely social reasons for a short time. Tenuous relationships within families can be destroyed if some relief is not given. The use of the term 'asylum' is perfectly respectable; it implies a benevolent institution affording shelter and support to some class of the afflicted. I accept that suitably staffed and managed hostels, crisis intervention teams and emergency clinics are relevant and very useful in this context, but we should also retain the facilities to admit patients as an alternative form of relief and care. There are also people who are inadequate and chronically impaired and need appropriate supportive environments, with protection from the stresses of life.

I continue to be struck by the change in some patients who move from acute admission wards to longer-stay wards. Whereas they showed marked disturbance on acute admission wards, where they were treated intensively by psychotherapists, psychologists and nurses, the pattern changed when in a quieter ward with a less demanding and more stable atmosphere. Space, time and tolerance are valuable attributes not easily found in compressed DGH units.

I feel that 'new' long-stay patients should be recognised as a significant group. One sees a small but important number of young people suffering from schizophrenia, with active, chronic symptoms which rarely abate and which cause intermittent severe disturbance. Patients with such problems can be contained in hospital reasonably well, and the challenge is always to provide a high standard of consistent care to maintain the abilities that remain. Patience is essential, to wait until the more psychotic elements have lessened and active rehabilitation can begin. This may take some years and, here again, a resource centre, or large hospital, can take a less frantic approach than a smaller DGH unit. An alternative placement for such patients could again be an establishment in the community. We know that Dr Douglas Bennett has such a hostel at the Maudsley Hospital. But this is near the hospital and, as has been pointed out, staffing levels are extremely high. So, to care for such patients properly and appropriately in a community, a significant clinical input of high quality nursing and medical staff is needed. One cannot think in terms of the usual local authority hostel. Another community focus is 'depot' clinics where regular injections of medication are given to schizophrenics. Such clinics can institutionalise patients as much as any hospital, and patients may be equally neglected in terms of medication and management.

John Reed has listed another problem of 'open door' policies: the inadequate chronic schizophrenic who drifts from the Embankment to prison, to hostels, to hospitals and to the street again but has no regular place to stay. It has been pointed out, somewhat cynically, that the decrease in the populations of the large psychiatric hospitals has been balanced by the increase in those of the prison hospitals.

An area for development is in primary care. Some four or five per cent of patients who go to GPs are referred to specialist mental illness services. A much larger proportion have some psychiatric illness and, of course, many more have psychological problems. Hence, there is scope for developing further services for the mentally ill, not only with professional help but, increasingly, with lay help. This raises the problem of relationships between professionals and voluntary workers. If you look at the 'Good Practices in Mental Health' reports (see bibliography) which a number of districts have prepared, it is always fascinating to see how this interaction occurs, with projects in hospitals being carried out by volunteers, with professionals working in the community advising self-help groups, or volunteers entirely running their own schemes.

To sum up, we need a comprehensive and flexible network of services - there is little disagreement about this. How do we implement changes? Medical superintendents can no longer determine rules and take strong action. We have multidisciplinary committees which take much time and can cripple any decision-making. Their success turns on goodwill, persistence, energy and impetus. While there can be so many frustrations in implementing quite basic plans in the community, we can take heart from the Hackney programme in its imaginative development of resources, and its success in coming to terms with planning restrictions and bureaucracy.

REFERENCES

Bewley T H, Bland M, Mechen D & Walch, E (1981). New
   Chronic Patients. <u>British Medical Journal</u>, 283,
   pp 1161-1164.
DHSS   (1975).   <u>Better Services for the Mentally Ill</u>.
   Cmnd 6233, HMSO, London.
Goldberg D & Huxley P (1980). <u>Mental Illness in the
   Community</u>. Tavistock, London.
Lomas G B G (1979). <u>Long-term Mental Illness in
   Hackney</u>. CPRU Working Note 1, Community Psychiatry
   Research Unit, Hackney Hospital.
NHS (1962). <u>Hospital Plan for England and Wales</u>.
   Cmnd 1604, HMSO, London.
Wing J K (ed) (1982). <u>Long-term Community Care:
   Experience in a London Borough</u>. Psychological
   Medicine, Monograph Supplement No 2, Cambridge
   University Press.

Chapter Eight

A HOUSE FOR ALL REASONS: THE ROLE OF HOUSING IN COMMUNITY CARE

Adrian Lovett

In this chapter I shall discuss what we have managed to achieve in Hackney by way of community provision, and indicate what could be achieved under ideal conditions. I shall try to identify some of the key elements in building up and maintaining a service, but shall not cover the clinical side, which is described in Chapter 7.

RESEARCH AND INFORMATION

Four years ago, in Hackney, information about the numbers of people needing any psychiatric service, let alone about the numbers needing specific types of psychiatric service, was virtually non-existent. As a housing worker, even one with a special interest in the subject and a willingness to try to contribute something practical, I had no definite idea of what was needed, where, or by whom.

The medical assessments of people on the council's waiting list for housing were of little use because mental illness, or 'nerves' as it was usually called, was given low priority compared to physical illness or disability. There was a quota of 60 to 70 lettings a year to rehouse people nominated by the social services department. But although we had many nominations for children and old people at risk, we received hardly any for people with problems due to mental illness. The priorities laid down for social workers put mental illness, together with mental handicap, so far down the list that very few people who were mentally ill were known to social services at all. The local health service was (and indeed still is) a huge bureaucracy that found it difficult to convey what sort of links it wanted with the local authority, and what sort of projects should be initiated.

A breakthrough came, not from within the health
service, but through charitable funding which
established the Community Psychiatry Research Unit
(CPRU) at Hackney Hospital. Their first task was to
identify the 'target' population. It was assumed
that those most likely to be helped by the
development of better community-based psychiatric
services were those people whose mental illness had
persisted for some time. These were defined as
people who had been inpatients on at least three
occasions during the current or previous year, or
who had had regular outpatient or drug treatment for
at least one year. All the hospital records were
checked and a cohort of 715 people with long-term
illness was identified - a sizable number to plan
for. In addition to demographic details, assessments
were made about medical needs, accommodation needs
and day-time occupation or employment needs.

In addition to providing the basic information
for the formulation of a programme to develop a
range of community facilities, the unit began to
break down the barriers between various somewhat
insular organisations by talking to many people
about what was needed and how any of it might be
achieved. In an ideal world, this information, and,
even more important, this attitude, would be a
routine part of the service in every health
district. Even in a world that is not ideal, it is
surprising, once you undertake a study of this kind,
how many people are willing to help, and how many
different sources of finance, including money from
trust funds and joint funding, may be available to
those who can find their way through their
complexities.

JOINT PLANNING

The second key element I have identified is the need
for a joint planning structure. I was lucky to be
invited to join a planning team which was already
very active, and whose members were prepared to
speak their minds. As well as a range of health
service staff it included representatives from the
local authority social services and housing
departments, the Community Health Council and
voluntary organisations. Merely getting the
representatives of different organisations together
does not amount to joint planning. That is an
altogether more ambitious exercise which requires
that participant organisations work together right
through the whole lengthy processes of planning and

implementation, and make a conscious and sustained effort to build in proper accountability to the democratic process of health and local authority decision-making. Having laboriously moved some way towards that in Hackney by March 1982, we had to start all over again within the re-organised NHS structure, and I estimate that this has set us back by anything up to a year. At the same time, central government thought fit to impose a reorganisation on Hackney's Housing Department, so that to our own 27,000 properties we were forcibly required to add a further 18,000 GLC properties. A double re-organisation of this kind would certainly not feature in my ideal world!

PHILOSOPHY

Ideally the joint planning body should have some cohesive philosophy. It need not be anything elaborate, but a requirement to make the even the baldest statement concentrates the mind, and an agreed statement is a valuable reassurance to fall back on when difficulties arise. Our own philosophy, such as it is, can be summed up in three short paragraphs:

1. Services provided for the mentally ill by the NHS, social services, housing and other bodies are interdependent; and therefore deficiencies in one will cause strains on the others. There will be an increasing need for a wide range of services in the community to supplement those offered by the health services.
2. The services provided should enable a person who is mentally ill to lead as normal a life as possible. In particular, admission to hospital should be limited to those persons for whom there is a clear indication of a need for a type of care which can only be given in a hospital setting.
3. Services should be as flexible and as local as possible, and should adapt to the clients' needs rather than forcing them to conform to an existing rigid structure.

This is obviously not the right answer for everyone. It can be modified and expanded, and the learning process of doing that, locally, in discussions which cut across individual service and professional boundaries, is every bit as important as the final statement itself.

BUILDINGS

The research study showed that although some patients had been in psychiatric wards for up to four years, there was no-one for whom their consultant thought this the most suitable provision. In order to act on this, and use hospital wards as, at most, a relatively short-stay provision, other types of buildings will be needed. We have identified a range of needs, which can be set out as a progression from the total dependence of the psychiatric ward through to the independence associated with an ordinary flat. Ideally there should be enough places at each point on the progression to enable people to move relatively quickly from one to another as their needs change. One solution to the problem of moving people from one building to another is to develop a system, as we have in Hackney, which moves the support rather than the client. The basic elements of our range of accommodation are ordinary council flats in which a person can be given more or less support (according to his/her needs at any time) by a multidisciplinary team of support workers from CPRU.

In addition to this accommodation there are a number of special projects which cater for specific needs:

1. Accommodation with a high level of support. A minimum of 20 places in accommodation with a great deal of day-to day support from a resident housekeeper, or maybe a couple, plus visiting community psychiatric nurses and occupational therapists, was thought necessary in order to provide permanent homes for those who would otherwise be in hospital or living in the community only with a very great amount of family support. So far one such scheme is being developed, which will have room for ten people. This scheme is making use of council property which we were unable to get through the project controls set by the Department of the Environment for sheltered housing for elderly people. We are now looking for another similar development in another part of the borough, in either council or housing association property.

2. Hostel type accommodation with less support. Hostel and communal accommodation of a variety of styles is needed for quite a large number of people with disabilities and chronic mental illness. Some should have a definite

rehabilitative approach, others should place
less emphasis on rehabilitation but provide a
tolerant and homely atmosphere, allowing residents to find a comfortable life-style
according to their individual capabilities. So
far we have definite plans for a communal home
for 24 people (in three groups of eight) in a
building being refurbished by London and
Quadrant Housing Trust in partnership with
Vanguard Commune. Until that is ready there are
two short-life schemes for up to 15 people. We
have had doubts about the large size of this
scheme, but the opportunity seemed too good to
turn down and care has been taken to ensure
future flexibility by designing it so that it
can be run as three separate units if required.
The only other places of this kind in the
borough are totally unsatisfactory commercial
'hotels' which do, however, provide a better
home than a park bench.

3. <u>Group homes and flatshares.</u> We provide for a
wide range of needs with absolutely standard
flats or houses, let to two or more people who
are able to give each other some mutual support
and company. The council has agreed to allocate
ten lettings a year for sharers nominated and
supported by the CPRU Support Network. We were
also able to offer a small block of ten 2-
person flats which we were unable to renovate
as standard housing units because of cut-backs
in housing capital allocations. The money for
renovation came from the North East Thames
Regional Health Authority and the block is
managed by the City and Hackney Association for
Mental Health. Four people live rent-free and
give social support to the other residents as
well as collecting the rents and having a
caretaking role. All costs, including the
nominal rent to the council are covered by the
weekly charge paid by residents, most of whom
live on supplementary or invalidity benefit.
After inevitable teething troubles in finding
compatible people, this scheme is now working
well. One interesting development is that a
young mentally handicapped man has moved in
and, as well as enjoying living independently
himself, seems to have something of a
stabilising influence on others.

4. <u>Cluster flats.</u> Our latest experiment is to try
to offer several flats on the same estate to
people who have been mentally ill. These flats

are scattered rather than concentrated, but are
within easy reach of each other. Initially
support services will be provided by CPRU in
collaboration with the staff of the local
social services hostel who will provide some
training in domestic skills as well as
continuing support for ex-hostel residents. In
the longer run we intend, with the help of
Tenants' Associations and local community
groups, to find friendly neighbours who are
able to provide low-key support through
informal social contact for which they would
get a small payment.
5. Independent living. In a borough with housing
problems as serious as those in Hackney, every
single letting, housing one person, probably
means that 19 or 20 others (who might have
accepted the flat) will have to wait even
longer. Although this may not seem an
auspicious time to promote rehousing on grounds
of mental illness, I think it is greatly to
Hackney Council's credit that they have
extended the medical priorities for people on
the waiting list to include schizophrenia as
one of the overriding priorities to qualify for
rehousing. Although numbers so far are small
they will certainly build up as the scheme
develops.

I feel that we need now to consolidate the
position we have reached, to monitor carefully the
various schemes as they come into operation, and to
be prepared to modify our policies and priorities in
the light of this knowledge and experience.
The basic meaning of the title of this paper,
'A House for all Reasons', is straightforward. There
are lots of reasons, or arguments, for using houses
rather than hospitals to provide homes for people
who are mentally ill, in particular:

- housing is (relatively) readily available;
- it gives a 'normal' environment which improves
  quality of life;
- it removes possible stigma, for people who
  currently live in what are seen to be institutions.

I was also trying to convey an echo of 'A Man
for all Seasons', that is an image of flexibility,
of an ability to adapt to changing circumstances in
a way that a psychiatric ward, and certainly a

psychiatric hospital, cannot. I did not, however, wish to imply that any rehousing should necessarily be in a house, rather than in a flat. Although I think that a house would be ideal, in Hackney, where over 85 per cent of council housing is in the form of form of flats on estates, it would be quite unrealistic to rule out the use of flats. I hope that my comments above, on the cluster flat scheme, have shown one practical and satisfactory way of using them.

ALTERNATIVE SOURCES OF HOUSING

There is a role for the housing authority, as well as for housing associations, to make available the accommodation for 'special' schemes such as those mentioned. The main reason, in Hackney, that we were able to persuade the council to use their own housing in this way was, ironically, that there were cuts in the capital allocation which resulted in there being vacant properties, unusable for standard housing purposes, and with no money for improvement work. It is important, in principle, for the local housing authority not to opt out of special schemes, not least because of the change in attitudes that it can bring about towards greater responsiveness to 'ordinary' housing and tenants. In our case it seems that schemes which came about for very practical reasons have worked well enough to instil confidence and gain more general acceptance amongst the council's members and officers.

Housing associations do, of course, have a great deal of experience and also the great advantage that, because of the manner in which they are funded, their schemes do not add to the authority's rate burden in the way local authority schemes do. Their smaller scale and greater autonomy also enable them to be more innovative than local authorities, and at times, more daring, in taking the calculated risks needed to establish new patterns of provision.

MANAGEMENT AND WELFARE

Buildings which are anything more than an individual flat have to be run by a management committee of some kind. Committees for the schemes mentioned above include people who work for the statutory services - health, social services and housing in particular. They also provide an opportunity to build up links between residents and the statutory

services. But essentially management of any such
project is the responsibility of voluntary
organisations, and in Hackney this has been a
problem. Until relatively recently there has been a
dearth of suitable voluntary agencies, and this
situation was exacerbated by the Council, which, in
the past, and in my view quite wrongly, equated a
low income area with a need to limit provision to
relatively low cost services. Out of this background
it has taken some time and a good deal of effort on
the part of intermediaries such as CPRU, whose role
is to motivate others into action, rather than
provide all the services themselves, to promote
voluntary agencies with a specialist interest in
mental health.

Those of us who are, in the main, concerned
with the non-medical elements of a service must
still remain aware of the priorities and constraints
faced by the medical services, so that the links
which enable a person to move easily between
facilities can be made and maintained. This awareness is also important in the context of making
changes to the system in response to changes in
clients' needs. If, for instance, someone is no
longer happy where he/she is living, there are two
immediate considerations: first, whether the
building and support services can be changed for the
better, and second, whether the person could move
elsewhere, if that is what they wish. The whole
question of support leads housing workers to
consider the problem of whether, and how far,
housing should have a welfare role. In practice, we
tend to expect other professionals to come to us
when our help is needed. We can make our presence
known through home helps, GPs, social clubs and
centres and then respond as best we can to requests.

This leads on to the role of social workers and
the whole social services department in the field of
mental illness. Whether it is generally true I am
not sure, but certainly in Hackney there is a
considerable clash of priorities, with children and
old people consistently being given much higher
priority than anyone with mental illness or
disability. When many referrals of this kind to
social services are met with a completely negative
response, we in the housing department have to
wonder whether we should, indeed, be trying to
provide support ourselves. Housing managers are now
not only helping people who were housed because they
were mentally ill, but also those who were rehoused
for other reasons, but have since become mentally

ill. In the past we experienced great difficulty in
dealing with such people, particularly on high
density estates, but where the community psychiatric
nursing (CPN) service has been involved, problems
with neighbours have diminished enormously. This, in
turn, has meant that the housing department has
become more willing to accept referrals in cases of
mental illness.

A related question is that of breaches of
confidentiality. If a housing manager becomes
worried about a tenant should the case be referred
to the CPN service or to social workers? How far
should a housing worker intervene? These are
questions to which I have no answer, but which are
becoming increasingly important in the context of
developing community services.

FUNDING

Obviously it would help to have more funds, but more
important than quantity is the flexibility with
which money can be used, especially that available
through joint funding arrangements. One valuable
improvement would be to have longer horizons. On the
housing front we do not know how much money has been
allocated to capital projects until far too late.
This is particularly frustrating for major capital
schemes which can take two or three years to develop
to the point of spending money, but which can get
nowhere without funding being guaranteed early on in
the process. The same is true for revenue, especially for the early years of a residential project
whilst income is being generated fairly slowly.

Many of the conditions attached to obtaining
funds from, for instance, the Housing Corporation,
the Department of the Environment/Inner Cities
Partnership programme, militate against providing
flexible and efficient forms of support. With such
funds staff are tied firmly to a particular project
or building even though a system based on a mobile
support team catering for a number of residents in
different types of accommodation has been shown to
work better.

So far in Hackney we have no experience of
joint, or even integrated operations, although we
have experience of joint planning. This is an area
which we need to develop, with constant monitoring
and feedback on successes and failures. As many
other contributors have said, it is very much a
question of attitudes on the part of the people
involved and of creating trust between members of

the different professions and between voluntary and
statutory agencies so that they can work efficiently
together to achieve agreed objectives.

CONCLUSION

A great deal remains to be done in Hackney, but I
hope this account will encourage everyone to review
the situation in their own area and see what more
can be done. If we can make progress in Hackney,
with all its problems, there must surely be a lot of
scope in other places!

DISCUSSION AND COMMENTS

Ian Diamant

Rather than presenting a critique of the statutory
sector I propose to contribute information about the
work of the voluntary sector, housing associations
in particular, in widening the range of supported
accommodation for vulnerable clients. I do not
believe that there is any conflict between the two
sources of housing, and in most instances they can
complement each other well.
   Housing associations have existed for far
longer than local authority housing. They date from
the almshouses of the sixteenth and seventeenth
centuries. There was a burst of development about
the turn of the century, with organisations like the
Guinness and Peabody Trusts who were large employers
needing to provide housing in the inner city for
their employees. However, local authority development was a major public sector housing
provision following the First World War, and
although housing associations started expanding in
the 1960s, it was not until the 1974 Housing Act,
which introduced a grant system called the Housing
Association Grant, that housing associations began
to have a significant effect on public sector
housing. In the period from the mid-1970s until the
Conservative Government's cuts took effect, housing
association ownership throughout the country doubled
from roughly a quarter of a million properties to
about half a million. The capital comes through two
sources. Approximately £6 million in 1982 came

through the Housing Corporation, an offshoot of the
Department of the Environment. Until the
Conservative Government came to power, half our
funding came from local authorities from their
Housing Investment Programme monies. This dried up
by last year, but is now picking up again. Housing
Association Grant on normal housing projects takes
care of about 80 per cent of the cost of each
scheme; about 20 per cent is paid in mortgages from
the money we receive in rents. I work as a special
projects officer, dealing with shared housing and
hostels. We tend to receive 100 per cent grants for
special schemes so we have no mortgage repayments -
a very artificial way of making our schemes seem
attractive to local authorities. This method of
funding has meant that a lot of local authorities
have supported us, not because of the work we do but
because it is financially advantageous for them.

Most of the 3,000 housing associations which
are registered with the Housing Corporation are also
registered charities. This number is slightly
deceptive, since only 500 do any actual housing
development and about 80 per cent of the money is
spent by only 50 or so of these. The reason for this
is that there are some associations which are large
and energetic, like London and Quadrant Housing
Trust, for which I work, and do a lot of general
family housing, as well as working in other areas:
housing for the elderly; housing for families;
special projects and work with specialist agencies.
There are large specialist associations like Anchor
(formerly Help the Aged), who provide housing for
the elderly and there are some which cater only for
small special groups - ex-servicemen, people who
work for British Airways. Associations differ
enormously in structure and in many ways are even
more diverse than local authorities. They also
differ in political outlook and in the way they
work.

Special project work really got off the ground
in 1977 with the Housing Corporation circular
relating to joint funding arrangements for caring
hostels. In a sense, this was an early version of
the idea of community care, recognising that housing
associations, with the experience of housing
development but still relatively small compared with
local authorities, could work in partnership with
other voluntary agencies and provide care as well as
accommodation. Although we talk in terms of
partnership, it is not a true partnership; we
appoint voluntary agencies as our agents to manage

properties on our behalf while we remain the
landlord. The residents are, therefore, licencees of
the housing association.
I must emphasise that our money comes from the
Department of the Environment and so is 'housing'
money. Personally, I do not recognise the divisions
laid down by the people who lend us the money, but
there are a number of things we cannot do. For
instance, we are not meant to involve ourselves in
Children's Homes and similar 'caring' schemes
considered by the social services departments and
the health service to be beyond our remit. Provision
defined as 'medium-care' by their standards is on
the border-line; one has to bend the rules a little
at times, so that housing associations do work on
low to medium-care types of schemes which are
normally of the social work nature. One further
constraint is that housing associations are not
allowed to do schemes in partnership with the
statutory sector. For instance, I cannot set up a
scheme directly with the probation services, but,
instead will work with a voluntary organisation
caring for ex-offenders. In Hackney we are
collaborating in this way with Vanguard Commune, a
voluntary organisation founded specifically to
enable special schemes for psychiatric patients to
be undertaken. Vanguard has members from the health
service, from the local authority and from CPRU, so
there are not many people who are working in a truly
voluntary capacity.
Adrian Lovett touched on the composition of
committees for special projects. There is a lot of
criticism about true voluntary committees because
often local people are not involved. For instance it
is almost always difficult to find a treasurer who
will examine the books for nothing and on time. In
the end we appoint someone and pay them, which is
what we should have done in the first place.
The real difficulties arise in relation to
revenue to run a project. Typically the rents we
obtain from the residents (usually from DHSS
payments and the housing benefits) cover about half
the running costs, and any project that employs
staff will require other monies to make up the
deficit. The financing of projects for the mentally
ill means going to local authorities since they
budget. However, it is often difficult for them to
make long-term commitments, because decisions about
the potential burden on local authorities in 10 to
15 years are affected by the reorganisation of the
health services and changes in joint funding.

Without a guaranteed source of funding for the
revenue deficit the Housing Corporation is reluctant
to approve the money for building or renovation
work. So again, rules have to be bent in order for
projects to get off the ground.

I was interested in Adrian Lovett's discussion
about different definitions of accommodation -
hostels, cluster flats, group homes. I have
completed a similar exercise in the housing
association movement; from January 1983 we have used
these terms. For us, the real issue is to do with
the type of management, and not the physical design
of the building. For example we organised a scheme
in a London borough, for homeless, rootless,
psychiatrically ill men, in their forties and
fifties. It was a fair-sized scheme providing
permanent housing for ten men with four double bedrooms, two single bedrooms, a living room, laundry
room, and an office. We convinced the planning
department that it was a single family dwelling.
Hence we did not need planning permission. When we
obtained a fire precaution certificate from the
environmental health department we agreed with them
that it was a house in multiple occupation. In order
to obtain revenue, the Housing Corporation agreed
that it was a hostel. The voluntary agency called it
a supportive group home. Some standardisation of
definitions is long overdue.

The size of schemes is a very interesting
issue, because housing associations have been
involved in special projects in a substantial way
only since 1977, and have, therefore, very little
experience of how successful their various schemes
are over a number of years. Our policy has been to
look for 30 or fewer bed-spaces, although there are
a few larger ones. You must remember that we are
closing down some very large institutions (of 500
and 1,000 beds) in London and replacing them with
smaller hostels and communal homes, so even when
talking about 100 beds it does seem rather a radical
change. We talked of 30 or fewer bed-spaces; the
number seems to be getting smaller by the week. I
suspect that my average now is about eight. Our
notion of a good size and style is small, shared
houses, of perhaps five persons, which have no
residential staff. Social work or other care staff
travel between several houses, which have common
management and are linked together for the purposes
of revenue budget. It seems that this is the way
that work for most housing associations is now
moving. There have, then, been some drastic changes

in the ideas about the style of supported housing
and these have been influenced by the type of social
work or caring element that was introduced into
housing association schemes because of the nature of
the partnership.
     I have painted something of a glossy picture of
the work of housing associations. A large percentage
of the money that housing associations now obtain
has come from our 'fair rent' family housing and is
being channelled into special projects. This has
been advantageous to us because such projects have
always been a difficult area of housing with
cumbersome and time-consuming procedures. Recently
we have established a number of sheltered projects,
(housing for the elderly is a good example), which
have become a significant part of our work. At the
beginning of 1982 a third of the public money going
into housing was spent by housing associations. Now
it is probably more than a third, because we have
been allocated money from the local authorities. We
have always been seen as innovators, supplementing
and filling in gaps in statutory housing provision,
but our role has been slowly changing to become
major providers. This change is potentially
dangerous because we have no statutory obligations
and therefore the provision we make will be
extremely patchy. We are not as accountable as a
local authority. We have no elected members since we
are managed by a management committee. I believe
that the voluntary sector must not see itself as the
major provider. We have a duty to defend the
statutory sector and make sure that there is
comprehensive provision, realising that the
voluntary sector has its part to play, can fill gaps
and is a useful place for experimentation.

Chapter Nine

PLANNING AN IDEAL SERVICE FOR NEWHAM: THE PROBLEMS

Deirdre Cunningham

This chapter describes the assessment of current
usage of psychiatric services in a London district
(Newham) with a view to planning a tailor-made
service in the district for the future.

Currently, all psychiatric beds are outside the
district, in Goodmayes Hospital in the neighbouring
district of Redbridge. A new nucleus hospital was
opened in Newham in 1982 with 300 beds, none of
which is for psychiatric use. Phase 2 of this
hospital, scheduled for completion in 1984, will
provide only maternity beds. However, the opening of
the nucleus hospital has changed the roles of
existing hospitals within the district, and in
consequence the buildings or sites of four of these
present hospitals will become available for alternative use by services such as psychiatry.

Assessments on which to base a description of
current use of the psychiatric service were made on
the basis of three parameters:

1. Assessment of current needs for services and
   comparison with usage data.
2. Projection of figures forward to 1991 with
   recommendations.
3. Assessment of measures which need to be taken
   to cope with any existing problems or with any
   reduction in services which implementation of a
   community-oriented system of care might entail.

ASSESSMENT OF CURRENT NEEDS FOR SERVICES AND
COMPARISON WITH USAGE DATA

Need was assessed using Bradshaw's taxonomy of need
(Bradshaw 1972), which identifies four categories:
   - normative need, i.e. as defined by a prof-
     essional;

- felt need, limited by the perceptions of the
  individual;
- expressed need or demand, i.e. felt need turned
  into the action of asking for a service;
- comparative need, where a measure is made of
  certain characteristics or conditions in a
  particular area or group who are receiving a
  service. If people with similar characteristics
  in another area or group are not receiving that
  service, then there is comparative need.

Normative Need
Norms for psychiatric services were derived from
Hospital Services for the Mentally Ill (1971), for
community psychiatric nurses from a 1980 DHSS
memorandum, for psychiatrists from the Royal College
of Psychiatrists' recommendations and for social
services provision for the mentally infirm from
Better Services for the Mentally Ill (DHSS 1975).
  It was apparent that, as a district, Newham has
marked over-provision of beds compared with the
numbers dictated by the guidelines. Newham has 85
per cent more beds than normatively required.
Equally worthy of note is Newham's lack of day
hospital places: only 18.4 per cent of the
recommended number are provided. Social services
provision of residential places meets the guidelines
and of day places exceeds the guidelines. Although
it appeared initially that there was a relative
shortage of community psychiatric nurses because of
their excessive workload, the workload was examined
in the light of preliminary results from this study
and has subsequently been cut down to approximately
the recommended figure.

Comparative Need
Newham was compared with five other districts in the
North East Thames Region to determine whether its
relative need tallied with its relative use. The
districts chosen were: Camden, City and Hackney,
Haringey, Islington and Tower Hamlets.
  When districts grouped in terms of relative
needs, as measured by social, socio-economic and
demographic variables (associated in the literature
with increased psychiatric morbidity) were compared
with districts grouped according to relative usage,
as measured by mean length of stay in psychiatric
beds and bed days per 1,000 population, no clear
relationship emerged. No district was included in
the 'low usage' group. Only one district, Camden,
was in the same 'need' group as 'usage' group.

Newham was unique in being in the relatively low
'need' group and in the relatively high 'usage'
group.
     Why was the usage so high in Newham? It was not
due to lack of social services provision. It was not
due to having too few community psychiatric nurses.
It was not due to the fact that every one of the
Newham residents who were admitted to psychiatric
beds went to hospitals outside the district. Nor was
the excessively long mean length of stay of Newham
residents compensated for by a low readmission rate:
Newham residents' readmission rate approximated the
regional average. Data collected for all hospitals
in North East Thames Regional Health Authority
suggest that high usage figures are a function of
type of hospital. Mean length of stay can be taken
to be a proxy for the proportion of 'old' long-stay
in a hospital and the proportion of 'old' long-stay
patients in Goodmayes Hospital, serving Newham,
appears to be the highest of all hospitals in the
region.
     By normative need, Newham is, therefore, over-
provided with beds (85 per cent too many) and under-
provided with day places (72 per cent too few). By
comparative need Newham is also over-provided with
beds.

Felt and Expressed Need
These were determined by:

     - administration of a questionnaire to all 108
       general practitioners;
     - administration of a questionnaire to the
       community psychiatric nurses and the day
       hospital psychiatric nurses;
     - interviews with the three psychiatrists
       responsible for Newham residents at Goodmayes
       Hospital;
     - interviews with the Director of Social
       Services, the chairman and secretary of the
       Community Health Council, and the secretary of
       Newham Mental Health Association (NMHA).

Only half the GPs and 63 per cent of the community
psychiatric nurses replied to the questionnaires, so
their responses have been used largely anecdotally.
     There were no suggestions that fewer beds were
needed. Not one group felt that an increase in the
number of day hospital places was a matter of any
priority. Whereas most GPs, NMHA and one
psychiatrist felt that top priority should be given

to moving acute beds to within Newham, the Community
Health Council's priority issue was that of moving
'old' long-stay beds to within the district with the
slogan 'Bring our Old Folks Back'. Two Goodmayes
psychiatrists would have preferred all beds to
remain at Goodmayes, regardless of DHSS or local
plans for developing community-based services. The
most important issue for the community psychiatric
nurses and especially for the day hospital psychiatric nurses was to have nurse management trained in
psychiatric nursing. Every one of the responses
mentioned this. The community psychiatric nurses
expressed as a further priority the need to increase
their own number. When the psychiatric nurses were
asked whether a crisis intervention team would
assist them with their work, 92 per cent said that
they thought that it would. However, only one
community nurse actually wished to be involved in
such a service, in contrast to all the day hospital
nurses.

Assessment of 'felt' and 'expressed' needs
highlighted certain aspects of the current service
which might be improved:

1. The Director of Social Services, the secretary
   of NMHA and the CHC all pointed to the lack of
   integration of the GPs with other psychiatric
   services. The community psychiatric nurses
   wanted greater liaison with the GPs.
2. The need for more jointly funded and/or
   interdisciplinary ventures between social
   services and health services was mentioned by
   the Director of Social Services, two psychiatrists and three GPs.
3. The need for an increased range of facilities
   in the community was mentioned by NMHA, one
   psychiatrist and three community psychiatric
   nurses.
4. The Director of Social Services suggested that
   patients should be in their own homes or in
   supported accommodation such as group homes
   rather than in hospital. Only one person, a
   community nurse, suggested that there should be
   a greater degree of liaison between health
   services and the housing department.

RECOMMENDATIONS FOR PROVISION OF SERVICES IN 1991

Numerical forecasts were made of provision for 1991
required to meet the guidelines for the expected
population of Newham (OPCS 1981). Newham's
considerable over-provision of beds according to

norms and compared with the other five districts has
not been justified on the grounds of 'need' in this
study but has been accounted for merely by the
availability of beds. Therefore it was not thought
necessary to provide more beds than the norms would
dictate for 1991. Although nobody in Newham seemed
to feel the need for more day places, it was not
thought desirable to fall short of government
guidelines for such provision for 1991. Cutting down
on beds for 1991 would mean that people who might
otherwise have expected to be resident in Goodmayes
Hospital in 1991 would be discharged and cared for
by means of community facilities. Whilst it is
feasible to envisage that many such people could
find (or be found) suitably supported accommodation,
it seems unrealistic, in the present employment
market, to suggest that they would find day-time
employment. They would need day-time occupation and
care and this could be provided by suitably run day
hospitals and day centres.

The normative predictions were, therefore,
modified in the light of the calculated needs for
services. A change of psychiatric policy towards
community-oriented services was assumed and
suggestions were made as to how to provide the
required beds using existing hospitals and sites
freed by the opening of the new nucleus hospital.
Suggestions were also made as to how to provide
alternative accommodation for the 'old' and the
'new' long-stay who may be discharged into the
community from the large psychiatric hospitals, and
for remedying some of the other problems highlighted
by the responses to the questionnaire. The
implications of the recommendations are that a
build-up of community services is essential.

REFERENCES

Bradshaw J A (1972). Taxonomy of Social Need, in
    Problems and Progress in Medical Care: Essays on
    Current Research. Seventh Series. Edited by G
    McLachlan. O.U.P. for Nuffield Provincial Hosp-
    itals Trust, London.
DHSS (1975). Better Services for the Mentally Ill.
    Cmnd 6233, HMSO, London.
Ministry of Health (1971). Circular HM(71)97.
OPCS (1981). Population Projections for England,
    1979-1991. Series PP3, No 4, HMSO, London.

Chapter Ten

FITTING THE JIGSAW TOGETHER

K A M Grant

Most of us would agree that services for the
'priority care groups' which include elderly people,
those with mental handicap and people with chronic
mental illness, should be improved. Most of us have
ideas about how improvements could be made. However,
often these ideas fail to get translated into
action.
    Let us consider how we might develop services
for a particular client group - long-term
psychiatric patients. First of all we must clarify
what the needs are. This necessitates identifying
both the expressed and unexpressed needs (and for
this a well-designed, easily accessible information
base as described in Chapter 2 is invaluable) for
the group as a whole. These needs are then
translated into ideas and proposals, primarily by
the professionals and others who are responsible for
providing care, and also, from time to time, by more
independent research agencies. Various activists -
local associations, the media, councillors, and,
naturally, patients and their close associates, will
also have a voice in asserting needs and in
proposing ways of satisfying them. In addition,
there will always be some unquantified needs to be
taken into account and allowed for.
    Ideas and proposals come in all shapes and
sizes, at all levels of sophistication and ranging
from the clearly essential to the wildly
impractical. One of my roles, as District Medical
Officer, is to take a hand in sorting out
priorities, both within the various care groups and,
more importantly, between them. I attempt to get the
various instigators of proposals to join forces
rather than compete, to agree on their own
priorities where possible, and I can give general
advice as to how to secure the most effective

package of results, given the needs that have been
demonstrated and the resources (always limited) with
which to satisfy them.

Many districts, and City and Hackney is a good
example, are unlikely ever to get their budgets
increased. If one looks very crudely at how the
health authority allocates its resources to meet
needs, it can be seen that there are usually serious
imbalances. The waiting time in City and Hackney,
for instance, to have a hernia treated is, on
average, four weeks. However, if you have a doubly
incontinent, demented, elderly relative, it would be
nearer two years before the NHS offered inpatient
support. With no new money coming in to build up
inadequate services, the health authority must look
for funds by reducing existing services in another
area of its work. What it is thereby doing is
evening out the inability to meet all the demands on
its financial resources.

The health service's record, however, in
cutting back some services in order to develop
others, is poor. When the City and East London Area
Health Authority was formed in 1974, its main
priority was to develop community and non-acute
services. In fact, at 1979 prices, out of a budget
of £120 million, the community budget increased by
some £200,000 (6 per cent) between 1974 and 1981.
This was in spite of the authority cutting back its
hospital bed numbers in the acute sector by a
quarter.

When it comes to trying to piece together the
parts of the jigsaw and come out with some equitable
division of resources one of the immediate problems
is the difficulty in finding out precisely where the
money goes in the NHS. The costing system is based
upon buildings rather than what happens within those
buildings. Thus it is at the present time difficult,
if not impossible, to find out how much is spent on
each client group, and what items and services that
money is spent on. We hope that specialty costing
will, in the future, tell us more accurately where
the money is going. Needless to say, this will not
necessarily mean that imbalances are any more likely
to be redressed, but it will make it easier to see
where the imbalance is and sort out longer-term
strategies.

A further problem is that the normal allies of
those interested in developing services for the
priority care groups, in particular the local
authorities and their members on district health
authorities, will often not accept a reduction in

any service at all, even if this is the only way to
release funds to improve the priority care group
services. This is seen as implementing unacceptable
cuts.

To return to our discussion of developing
services: in spite of the problems mentioned, it is
possible to achieve some changes. However, in
translating ideas and proposals into plans and a
programme for action, there are a number of hazards.
It is obviously essential that the professionals who
are preparing the proposals understand the planning
system. But because of the way budgeting is done the
people who are preparing the plans are not given
budgets to work to so they are not able to assess
the likelihood of funding. In consequence, planning
for the different care groups is, apart from
intervention by someone like myself, completely
blind. Finally, because of the way the service is
organised, all plans must be submitted to, and
approved by, at least two authorities. In theory,
proposals for health authority developments are sent
to the District Management Team who co-ordinate a
package for the district and submit it to the
District Health Authority members for approval. In a
similar manner, proposals relating to local
authority developments progress through steering
groups, and approval is sought from members of the
appropriate local authority committees.

In addition to these two routes for proposals,
there is the possibility of joint financing of
projects which fall within the statutory
responsibilities of both local authority and health
service. At present, the joint finance system is
superimposed on the other planning and financing
systems: proposals go first to the District Joint
Care Planning Team, which has members from both
authorities, and then to the Joint Consultative
Committee for approval. The different systems for
getting proposals approved and funded tend to
militate against collaborative efforts and co-
ordinated programmes, especially for groups like
those with chronic mental illness where movement
between health service and local authority (and
perhaps voluntary) facilities is unpredictable, but
should be flexible. Proposals tend to come without
any strategic character. A further deficiency of
this disjointed system is that resources are often
used in a non-profitable way and there may be
difficulties in incorporating projects using 'soft'
money (for instance from charitable sources) into
mainline funding. The introduction of more

widespread joint planning systems, not restricted to
joint finance money, would certainly improve
flexibility and efficiency for planning and for the
resultant services.
     Within the City and Hackney Health Authority we
have set up a joint planning system based on care
groups (the planning teams mentioned by Adrian
Lovett in Chapter 8) for the elderly, elderly
mentally ill, mentally handicapped and the mentally
ill. The function of these groups is not just to
suggest how to spend joint finance money, but also
to make joint plans for the longer-term development
of services for each client group. In addition, when
setting budgets we 'top-slice' £1 million off the
total for the district to be spent on services for
the priority care groups and community health
services. Only after this amount has been reserved
do we set the budgets and assess what can be
afforded for the acute services. Probably this
method of labelling money for specific services is
the only way in which improvements to non-acute and
community services can be ensured.
     There are one or two pieces of advice which I
would offer to those who aspire to get their ideas
translated into practice. It is important to avoid
spending time on projects which, however worthy in
themselves, have no chance of getting money in the
context of the whole district (or regional) service.
When we are considering the priority care groups it
is essential to understand the planning systems of
the two statutory authorities and also how voluntary
organisations operate. All planning systems are
cumbersome and time-consuming, but frustrations can
be minimised by understanding the timetables of the
different authorities and respecting their
deadlines. Judicious pressure, when there is a good
case, applied to the appropriate person within the
authority concerned can be helpful. In the health
authority it is the officers who effectively make
the choices and decisions, whereas in the local
authority there is much more member involvement.
Lobbying is important, not just to get proposals
through the appropriate planning groups, but to make
sure that, if possible, there is an advocate at a
high level. Finally, it is useful for those of us
who have to sort out priorities and undertake
strategic planning, to have advance notice of any
substantial developments which can be foreseen, so
that steps can be taken to reserve funds.

Chapter Eleven

THE NURSING ELEMENT IN AN IDEAL SERVICE

Paul G Beard

Community psychiatric nursing began about 28 years
ago mainly as a result of the drug revolution,
particularly the phenothiazine group. At that time
it was very much linked to the administration and
the supervision of drugs and the surveillance of
patients suffering from schizophrenia.

During the last decade rapid growth, both in
the number and size of services, has occurred. In
1981 the Community Psychiatric Nurses Association
(CPNA) published a survey showing that there were
1,716 community psychiatric nurses (CPNs) in over
200 centres throughout the UK, 50 per cent of which
were not located in hospitals. Expansion has
continued since then, though perhaps less rapidly.
Now most if not all districts in the UK have a CPN
service with an operational base within the
district, or have access to one. This is less true
in the field of mental handicap although this
speciality is expanding also.

The first question one should ask is: what do
community psychiatric nurses do? Apart from broad
outline accounts little attempt to date has been
made to describe and evaluate the work of the CPN or
to measure intervention outcomes. So in building up
a CPN service one cannot be certain of the exact
effect it will have on a given population. In
practice the role of the CPN is diverse and varies
from district to district. Parnell (1977) in her
study of community psychiatric nurses described
where people worked, and the practical elements of
their role. Sladden (1979) highlighted the
involvement with medication. Since the early 1970s
evaluative studies such as Warren (1971), Leopoldt
et al. (1974), Harker et al. (1976), Corrigan & Soni
(1976), Hunter (1978), and Paykel et al. (1982) have
emerged but methodological problems have primarily

been responsible for what is still a poorly evaluated yet developing area of mental health nursing.

Two other books which I consider to be the handbooks of community psychiatric nursing are Carr et al. (1980) **Community Psychiatric Nursing** and Butterworth & Skidmore (1981) **Caring for the Mentally Ill in the Community.** In my own article, 'Community Psychiatric Nursing - A Challenging Role in 1980' (Beard 1980), I briefly described an organisational and nursing practice framework detailing some of the possibilities and ideas for future development. In that article, I listed almost all the various forms of practice that nurses could undertake, but I did not imply that all nurses should actually undertake the full range (for example, group work, individual psychotherapy, counselling, behaviour therapy, and so on). Nursing practice should relate to the skills and training of an individual nurse. One cannot assume that because a nurse has the Registered Mental Nurse qualification that he/she can instantly undertake such a wide range of therapies. The Joint Board of Clinical Nursing Studies course in community psychiatric nursing places an emphasis on educating nurses, as opposed to training them. The course enables them to examine role and function and prepares them to be better managers of their time, for example in handling a case load. But it does not actually train them to be therapists. The acquisition of such skills may present major problems for those districts where there is little or no commitment, financial or otherwise, to on-going education and training for nurses. Apart from post basic training, nurses should consider trainings which do not lead to a specific nursing qualification, for example counselling courses. The completion of such training should lead to a period of refinement and incorporate supervision. The work of the CPN is diverse and management needs to understand it as such if nurses are to feel supported in their work.

Carr et al. (1979) talked about the various aspects of the CPN: the nurse therapist, the nurse educator, the nurse manager, the nurse clinician and the nurse consultant. The management of nursing practice is an important issue, both inside and outside the hospital. Management has a res-ponsibility to keep abreast of the developments in nursing practice and to ensure that varying flexible levels of help and support are available.

Sladdon (1979) states that the CPN 'has the ability to operate within the medical, social and the psychological frame of reference, which distinguishes him or her from other workers'. This overlap with other disciplines can be a problem, with obvious disadvantages to the client, so there should be a commitment at organisational level to bring fieldworkers from the various disciplines together, by encouraging shared learning for shared care. If an organisation is committed to the disciplines working together, then the staff will see each other as facilitators of an effective and co-ordinated plan for a particular family or patient. A community nurse and a social worker may be able to discuss which is the best worker for a case, not necessarily solely on the grounds of the presenting problem fitting neatly into one or other's background. One of those workers may already be established with a family or patient. If the nurse is well established, and the problems are of a social nature, the nurse could still have key-worker responsibility, perhaps with supervision from, and certainly in close touch with, the social worker. Workers from different disciplines should be able to work supportively together and share responsibility, but recognition from the relevant professional organisations is essential.

Let us move on to the questions of reponsibility, accountability and supervision. Work accountability is perhaps the most thorny issue. Services which operate closed referral systems and additionally are inappropriately monitored by nursing management more often than not perpetuate a line of work accountability to the consultant psychiatrist. So in effect the psychiatrist may be prescribing nursing intervention. I disagree with this. Accountability should be to the nurse manager, provided that he or she is suitably experienced and equipped to supervise and monitor community nursing activity. This should not imply that the CPN should not report to the consultant on the patients under his/her charge. Supervision is something often misunderstood and feared by nurses, but sensibly used it can support, stretch and strengthen the nurse in the practice of nursing, gaining insight and skills on an incremental basis. Supervision can facilitate a more objective approach to the assessment and delivery of care. In my own district CPNs use peer group supervision successfully and although they can call upon me to discuss any particular case there is no expectation that I am an

'expert'. In certain situations nurses are
encouraged to consult someone from another
discipline who does have the necessary skills, as
long as the lines of accountability are understood
and remain with the nurse manager.

No less important are the models and the
philosophies surrounding the community psychiatric
nursing service or indeed the nursing contribution
in any district to mental health care. It is
appropriate to mention training here again, because
I would like to see many more opportunities in the
future for multi-professional learning. The
acquisition of skills and the ability to respond
flexibly to the patients and community are central
to the successful development of alternatives in
mental health services. Managers have a key part to
play in facilitating change and in enabling staff to
exploit their potential. Practitioners and managers
can together promote innovative developments. I am
concerned that as of yet, the cost implications of
locally-based mental health services have not been
fully realised, particularly by government. The
challenges of tomorrow depend not only on cash but
on the preparation of existing staff to grasp the
challenge and move forward with confidence. Retraining, and a process of attitudinal change must
commence now. Moreover, basic nurse training must
incorporate concepts contingent with the emergence
of new patterns of service.

The contribution of the nursing service is
variable. In districts where the nursing service is
strong, backed by nurses who can vocalise their
patients' needs, articulate their contributions and
gain the respect of their colleagues, initiatives
other than medical ones are possible. The presence
or otherwise of an 'open' referral system to the CPN
service is a useful indicator to gauge the level of
nursing activity in planning and implementing a
flexible range of services. The development of
locally-based services should be properly evaluated
so that the increased funding which I believe the
services will command can at least be defended with
factual evidence to demonstrate their value.
Planning ultimately involves normatives which serve
as a guide to staffing levels, but which can also be
very misleading. Obviously, one needs to consider
geographical location and special local needs. For
example, in a compact urban district time spent
travelling may be much less than in a rural district
where patients might live 50 miles apart. Staffing
levels depend also on the basic approach and

philosophy adopted. If an 'open' referral system
operates, where community nurses are responsible for
preparing the community for the acceptance of mental
illness and mental disturbance within the community,
and if nurses are seen as agents of early detection
working closely with psychiatrists, primary care
teams (including general practitioners), social
services and voluntary organisations, then higher
staffing ratios are required than for a service that
will simply receive referrals previously assessed by
a psychiatrist. About 95 per cent of people who
attend general practice with emotional disturbances
are not seen by psychiatrists. Some of this 95 per
cent go to their doctor as a consequence of life
events or life crises which will respond to short-
term intervention and/or practical help. Where there
are good links with primary care services one is
likely to get to know about family or individual
'breakdown' early on.

Nursing should be seen in the context of its
contribution as one of the elements in an ideal
service. One could gradually build up a team of
able, self-motivated and dynamic nurses but if the
team has to work in isolation from kindred
disciplines the nursing impetus could be diluted
since many families/patients require the shared
responses and skills of several disciplines. I think
there is every reason to feel encouraged by the
'Care in the Community' initiative (see references
in Chapter 1), designed to promote schemes to care,
in the community, for people who would otherwise
remain in long-stay wards in large mental hospitals.
I believe that the health service can legitimately
take the lead since many of the skills needed lie
within its sphere. For instance, if we are trying to
establish units of accommodation in the community
for chronically ill or disabled patients, few
disciplines other than nurses have, through
experience, learned to respond to chronicity,
although nursing care alone may sometimes lack the
imagination such projects require.

The organisation of community psychiatric
nursing services is the topic on which I wish to
finish. Before the most recent re-organisation there
was a distinct difference in the way the CPN service
was managed in what is now the Bloomsbury Health
District. Bloomsbury was an amalgamation of the
former South Camden District of Camden and Islington
Area Health Authority, and the North East District
of Kensington and Chelsea and Westminster Area
Health Authority. In South Camden the CPN service

was managed by the community division, and in the
North East District by the psychiatric division. In
many respects the philosophies of the two component
parts were very similar; the differences were most
noticeable at managerial level. In the new structure
the service is managed by an Assistant Director of
Nursing Services (Community Mental Health),
accountable to the DNS (Mental Health). The outcome
of this change will, I believe, depend on several
key issues being realised: the need for the
community unit and the mental health unit to work
closely together, the former continuing to accommodate some CPNs in health clinics and centres;
the need for a well-organised support system for
fieldwork staff, including peer group supervision
and active staff development programmes geared to
meet the needs of each individual member of staff;
the need to ensure that those CPNs based in health
centres and clinics do not become professionally
isolated from their mental health nursing
colleagues, and the need to ensure that hospital-
based CPNs clearly identify their roles in relation
to the needs of the local population in promoting
early detection as well as tertiary care.

Finally, it is, in my opinion, imperative that
community psychiatric nursing services are organised
on a district-wide basis, spearheaded by a suitably
trained and experienced nurse manager, with a good
understanding of community mental health and social
concepts and ideas. I am not advocating that all
CPNs should be based in one centre, but that there
should be some corporate identity. It is
professionally unacceptable to disperse or
distribute CPNs throughout a district, attaching
them to a variety of clinical teams (with the
implication that the nurse is accountable to the
senior nurse in that location) unless each CPN has
in-depth and practical experience of nursing in the
community. Monitoring and managing community nursing
services is different from managing ward-based
nursing; it should be recognised as such and given
the level of professional expertise it deserves.

REFERENCES

Beard P G (1980). Community Psychiatric Nursing - A Challenging Role. Nursing Focus, 1, 8, pp 306-307.

Butterworth C A & Skidmore D (1981). Caring for the Mentally Ill in the Community. Croom Helm, London.

Carr P J , Butterworth C A & Hodges B E (1980). Community Psychiatric Nursing. Churchill Livingstone, Edinburgh.

Community Psychiatric Nurses Association (1980). National Survey of Community Psychiatric Nursing Services. Report R8007.

Corrigan J & Soni S (1977). Community Psychiatric Nursing: an Appraisal of its Impact on Community Psychiatry in Manchester. Journal of Advanced Nursing, 2, pp 347-354.

Harker P, Leopoldt H & Robinson J R (1976). Attaching Community Psychiatric Nurses in General Practice. Journal of the Royal College of General Practitioners, 26, 170, pp 666-671.

Hunter P (1978). Schizophrenia and Community Psychiatric Nursing. National Schizophrenia Fellowship.

Joint Board of Clinical Nursing Studies. Nursing the Mentally Ill in the Community (Community Psychiatric Nursing). JBCNS Course 810.

Leopoldt H, Hopkins H & Overall R (1974). A Critical Review of Experimental Nurse Attachment in Oxford. Practice Team, 39, 2 pp 4-6.

Parnell J W (1977). Community Psychiatric Nurses. A Descriptive Study. The Queen's Nursing Institute.

Paykel E S, Mangan S R, Griffith J H & Burns T P (1982). Community Psychiatric Nursing for Neurotic Patients: A Controlled Trial. British Journal of Psychiatry, 140, pp 573-581.

Sladden S (1979). Psychiatric Nursing in the Community. Churchill Livingstone, Edinburgh.

Warren J (1971). Long-acting Phenothiazine Injections given by Psychiatric Nurses in the Community. Nursing Times, 67, pp 141-143.

Chapter Twelve

PLANNING A PSYCHIATRIC INTENSIVE CARE UNIT

Ruth Seifert

INTRODUCTION

For the last 20 years or so, there has been growing concern about the care of psychiatric patients who need a degree of security for their treatment and management. Before the nineteenth century, 'lunatics' who were convicted of a felony or who were dangerous were sent to the local gaol and became objects of derision and amusement to the public, but otherwise were grossly neglected. In 1863 Broadmoor opened as the first of what are now the 'special hospitals', whose purpose is to admit and treat patients with criminal, violent or dangerous tendencies, on compulsory orders under conditions of special security. Ordinary psychiatric patients were accommodated in mental hospitals or psychiatric units, most of which, prior to 1959, had locked wards. Offenders and difficult non-offenders could usually be managed, and nursing and medical staff had considerable skill in their care, although conditions and methods were sometimes questionable. The movement towards unlocking doors and community-oriented care, with the provisions of the 1959 Mental Health Act, meant that patients presenting special management problems and requiring secure accommodation, but not to the level of the special hospitals, could no longer be easily accommodated in existing wards. The Working Party on special hospitals reported in 1961 (Ministry of Health 1961) and identified a need for 'special diagnostic centres', providing an intermediary function between the special hospitals and the NHS services. Only one such centre materialised. The Committee on Mentally Abnormal Offenders (the Butler Committee) was appointed in 1972 to review the law and the services. In 1974 the committee issued an interim report recommending the provision of regional secure units in the NHS as a matter of urgency. Patients were frequently inappropriately placed, or detained longer than necessary in prisons and special hospitals or accommodated without sufficient care in ordinary psychiatric wards. An initial target of 2,000 secure places was suggested by Butler. At the same time, the revised report of the DHSS Working Party on security in NHS psychiatric hospitals (the Glancy Report) (DHSS 1974) recognised a need for secure units for a small proportion of the psychiatric hospital population, and recommended that 1,000 beds would be required for England and Wales. A direct supplementary financial allocation from DHSS to the Regions was set up, followed in 1975 by design guidelines (DHSS 1975) and advice to each Regional Health Authority (RHA) to draw up plans for regional secure units for the treatment of seriously mentally disturbed people, some of whom might also be offenders.

The final report of the Butler Committee (DHSS et al. 1975) expressed its disappointment and concern that no progress had been made in establishing the units, feeling that the lack of interim funding was one important reason. In 1976, then, a special recurring revenue allocation was made to each region to be used to provide interim secure accommodation until proper units could be established. Since then, some RHAs have set up planning teams and a few 'interim' units have been established.

The North East Thames Regional Health Authority reviewed their policy in May 1980 in the light of continued lack of progress in developing facilities for psychiatric intensive care, and agreed that a network of psychiatric intensive care units (PICUs) should be established throughout the region, each operating independently for an agreed catchment area. At a subsequent meeting the City and Hackney District, having indicated an interest in setting up a PICU at Hackney Hospital, was asked to take responsibility for preparing details of the scheme. A Working Party was set up, and I, as a consultant psychiatrist with an interest in forensic psychiatry, have been closely involved in planning and may, in due course, run the unit.

'SECURE' OR 'INTENSIVE CARE'

The RHA's original idea was to have interim or medium secure units, similar to those in South

London, where the main unit is at Bethlem Hospital with a linked interim/medium secure unit at Tooting Bec Hospital. From my experience it seems that such units are quite inadequate as a means of improving the care for severely disturbed patients since they are usually not purpose built, but are ordinary wards converted to provide security. In practice, as the consultant would agree, the medium secure unit has become just another locked facility, retaining patients for whom there is little hope of rehabilitation. We have, therefore, explored carefully the principles for our own unit; these are best described by the name psychiatric intensive care unit. The unit will provide intensive care and treatment, for mentally ill people living in the London boroughs of Newham, Tower Hamlets and Hackney, including those who have exhibited disturbed and disruptive behaviour which makes them difficult to manage on an acute ward. The aim will be to provide a level and style of care so that within an average of six to ten months a patient can be discharged either to an ordinary psychiatric ward or to the community on an outpatient basis. The unit will provide conditions of security though not necessarily by means of locking doors. Security will be achieved by a high level of staffing with specially trained staff who can maintain constant observation of all patients and carry out planned programmes of therapeutic activity. Security devices will be kept to a minimum to avoid creating an institutional or prison-like atmosphere which we do not feel likely to be conducive to improving general confidence and trust.

CATEGORIES OF PATIENTS

It is difficult, in view of the dearth of systematic information, to state precisely which patients need increased care of the kind envisaged in the PICU. The enquiry conducted by the Royal College of Psychiatrists (1981) identified two principal groups of patients:

1. Those who are persistently aggressive and repeatedly try to get out of hospital. Patients such as these can cause extreme distress to other patients if treated on an open general ward and may lead to others, who are equally ill, discharging themselves prematurely.
2. Those who may be labelled 'socially disabled', often with no clear psychiatric diagnosis. In

the past such patients have stayed for long periods in institutions, but increased community care has demonstrated that although such 'asylum' may relieve problems for society and the individual for a short time, it is not a long-term solution.

The Royal College report (p 8) continues:
The problem of providing adequate care for these categories of patients has been made worse by the emphasis placed on the needs of 'mentally disordered offenders'. These offenders often come within one or other of the two groups (above), who show a degree of disturbance that is very similar to the non-offenders and present similar problems of management. Many other offenders, however, show very little behavioural disturbance and their offences may be trivial events such as petty shop-lifting or the theft of milk from doorsteps. Whether a patient presents as an offender or not is usually more a question of chance. The great majority of mentally disordered offenders can be managed adequately within a short-stay community-based inpatient facility, usually in an open-door environment, and open beds should continue to be available for them.

ESTIMATES OF NEED

One of the great problems in preparing the detailed plans for our PICU has been the difficulty in obtaining information about the total numbers of people who might need intensive care. For some time I have been trying to obtain information about how many mentally ill people are in prison. It has proved possible to get figures from the special hospitals but so far I have not succeeded in discovering how many Hackney residents are currently serving prison sentences and in need of treatment for mental illness. The government does not know how many prison inmates are receiving, or require, such treatment, although the Home Office has made several attempts, based on the returns from medical officers which use the crude diagnostic criteria of the Mental Health Act categories of mental disorder, to estimate the number of individuals in prisons who should appropriately be in a hospital setting. It seems clear that until some PICUs are actually opened no-one is in a position to undertake the research which will answer questions of this sort.

PLANNING CONSIDERATIONS

Security

Physical security devices will be unobtrusive and the emphasis will be on high staffing levels, with experienced staff, and constant supervision. Safety features will be incorporated into the design to achieve a secure 'envelope' and will include supervision of movement into and out of the unit by means of electro-mechanical control of the entrance. There will be a night observation station with audio-visual interconnection with the staff room; windows will be designed with small panes to prevent entrance and exit.

Size

It has been difficult to estimate the number of places needed for this catchment area of about 550,000 people. However, using the most usually accepted norm, that from the Glancy Report (DHSS 1974), of 20 beds per million population, then a total of 11 beds would be required. This figure has been increased to 12 to allow for the fact that the PICU we are planning has to cater for one of the more deprived inner city areas of the country.

Site

We have been anxious to ensure that such an important development to us, and indeed a model for others, should be properly sited. Regional policy stated that units should be provided by converting existing accommodation. We therefore considered in great detail the possibility of converting wards on two hospital sites, with five alternatives in mind. It is important to have the PICU on a general hospital site in order to maintain links with all other services, including general acute psychiatry. Our conclusion, after much deliberation, was that there should be a new structure (above the psychiatric day hospital in fact) which would have all the advantages of a purpose built design for its specialised function.

Since the original plans were prepared, ideas about the siting of the unit have altered. It will now probably be a free-standing, two-storey building placed in conjunction with existing psychiatric wards and sharing occupational therapy facilities and the gardens when suitable.

Staffing

It is fundamental to the philosophy and objectives of the unit that the staffing ratios should allow for constant supervision to anticipate and prevent violent episodes where possible and to contain them if they occur. There will also be an intensive programme of therapy designed to suit the needs of each individual in the unit. This is an inner city PICU (the first), surrounded by a densely populated residential area and with no large, secure, recreational area. Imaginative use will be made of existing sports and recreational facilities. Again, a high staffing ratio will be important. The unit will have a consultant psychiatrist in charge, with fully trained nurses, psychologists, occupational therapists and a social worker. There will also be a registrar and a senior registrar who will be engaged in research. Although each discipline will have primary responsibility for certain activities specific to their own specialty, the emphasis will be on multidisciplinary care, and all staff will be involved in all the activities of the unit. Our intention is that experience at all levels on the unit will be incorporated into training schemes in each discipline.

RELATIONSHIP TO OTHER FACILITIES

A common factor linking all admissions, from whatever source, will be that the patient's usual home is within the catchment area of Newham, Tower Hamlets and City and Hackney. The unit will accept referrals from a variety of sources around the country: directly from courts, prisons or youth treatment centres; from special hospitals where patients have been inappropriately placed because of lack of facilities in the NHS. Patients may also be accepted from special hositals as the first step in rehabilitation, or from acute wards where they have become particularly disturbed. We also intend to try to improve relationships between referring agencies and the staff of the unit. Patients will be assessed by a multidisciplinary group of staff before admission to ensure that they have the potential to benefit from the intensive care offered.

It is not anticipated that most patients will remain in the unit for more than about six months, although some may remain longer. Following a discharge and placement conference most patients will move to the general psychiatric services, either as inpatients on an acute ward or as day

patients. PICU staff will be involved in follow-up
and aftercare to ensure that there is a continuity
in style of care and that progress is maintained. A
range of supported accommodation, from a medium-stay
hostel to permanent local authority shared flats, is
available or being developed for people leaving the
unit who cannot or do not wish to return to their
previous home. We do not feel that, in our district
at least, it is either desirable or necessary to
have hostels specifically linked with the PICU,
since integration into the standard community
facilities will improve chances for rehabilitation.
Because we have been able to include a research post
in the team to staff the PICU we will be able to
monitor the use made of the unit, with continuing
research into the community and social needs of
patients who are discharged. Resources will be
channelled into such projects as necessary in order
to minimise the relapse rate, and we hope that our
findings will enable other districts to plan their
own facilities with more confidence.

REFERENCES

Committee on Mentally Abnormal Offenders (1974).
    Interim Report. Cmnd 5698, HMSO, London.
DHSS (1974). Revised Report of the Working Party on
    Security in NHS Psychiatric Hospitals (Chairman,
    Dr J Glancy). HMSO, London.
DHSS (1975). Regional Secure Unit Design Guidelines.
    DHSS.
DHSS, Home Office, Lord Chancellor's Office (1975).
    Report of the Committee on Mentally Abnormal
    Offenders (Chairman, Lord Butler of Saffron Walden
    K G), Cmnd 6244, HMSO, London.
Ministry of Health (1961). Special Hospitals: Report
    of a Working Party. HMSO, London.
The Royal College of Psychiatrists (1980). Secure
    Facilities for Psychiatric Patients. A Comp-
    rehensive Policy. Unpublished.

Chapter Thirteen

THE GENTLE TOUCH: PRINCIPLES FOR PROGRESS

Gillian Lomas

The realistic historian would argue that much far-
reaching change stems from serendipity - the happy
accident that puts resources, circumstances and
people together to spark off a chain of events. What
is happening in the City and Hackney Health
District, and with luck in others, is just such a
phenomenon. For those of us involved, our main claim
is in recognising the signs and omens and in being
prepared to grasp both the certainties and the
straws. This chapter recounts some of what we now
recognise as necessary, if not sufficient,
preconditions; expounds the principles upon which
our community services are being planned and built
and touches on one or two of the more tangible
successes. Our intention is always to try the
gentle, subtle ways of effecting changes, to graft
new services on to the better parts of existing ones
and to integrate old and new.
     First a brief description of what is taking
place and planned. Since 1974 there has been no
access to long-stay psychiatric beds (previously
available in Long Grove Hospital, Epsom) for City
and Hackney patients, and virtually all adult
general psychiatric illness has been treated in the
district general hospital unit, which had beds for
acute adult psychiatry, an emergency service, a
small number of community nurses, outpatient clinics
and day hospital facilities.
     By 1977 the system was uncomfortably silted up,
to a great extent by readmissions of patients whose
illness had a substantial social component, the
'non-copers' with inadequate statutory or personal
support networks, and by patients with chronic
illness or disability, for whom full hospital care
was not the most desirable solution. Various unco-
ordinated attempts were being made - in traditional

ways - to provide alternatives to hospital for these
patients; these were dogged by lack of a clear
notion of the numbers and circumstances of people
needing extra help. A six-month statistical study,
financed by the Mental Health Foundation and the
Gatsby Trust, identified the long-term population
and assessed its needs in order to provide the basis
for a programme for action to fill part of the gap.
This programme covered a range of housing,
employment and social projects, as well as
continuing research, meshing with the planned and
existing hospital-based services. The basis upon
which this programme was drawn up and executed is
discussed below.

The Community Psychiatry Research Unit came
into formal existence in 1979 and has, since then,
worked with the District Planning Team for Mental
Illness to stimulate progress, and implement the
planned programme of action.

WHAT CHANGES WERE NEEDED?

It was fairly clear, several years ago, that there
were two main areas for improvement. Firstly, the
range of facilities was inadequate, and secondly
there tended to be constant eruptions and
bottlenecks when it came to developing new elements
of the service.

In most districts there are perfectly well
developed psychiatric services; there are social
services; there is a housing department; there are
usually some voluntary agencies with an interest in
mental health. What is most often missing is the
means of co-ordinating the planning processes and
the activities of these agencies. Inevitably there
are gaps between them. Even if there are not actual
gaps in the service that is provided, there are
difficulties at the interfaces, both within
organisations and certainly between them.

Our aims, therefore, have been to expand
facilities to cover the full range of needs (insofar
as these are identified and understood - in itself
another problem) and to take responsibility for
acting at the interfaces between agencies to try to
ensure 'smooth' access to, and pathways between, the
different parts of the service, so that the
difficulties of the transfer from being 'patient' to
becoming 'client' and returning to being an
'ordinary (well) person' are coped with by those
giving the care, rather than by those receiving it.

ACHIEVEMENTS

There have been changes of three kinds:

1. Increase in range of facilities and services, such as:

   - better psychiatric emergency service
   - more community psychiatric nurses
   - more beds and day care for psychogeriatrics
   - CPRU Support Network with accommodation
   - a specialist clinician in community psychiatry
   - City and Hackney Association for Mental Health
   - Vanguard Commune, managing accommodation
   - Industrial Education Unit run by the Psychiatric Rehabilitation Association.

2. More communication and co-ordination at practical level, such as:

   - project management teams meeting regularly - psychiatrists, housing association officers, social workers, CPRU staff, residents etc.
   - medical students, nurses and other staff involved with voluntary projects
   - referrals and queries in connection with council housing transfers and housing welfare problems
   - joint development of schemes.

3. More attention to long-term strategy and preliminary research:

   - information to hand to prepare strategic proposals for 10-year plan
   - stream of research and action projects at various stages of development
   - planning for psychiatric services in connection with new Homerton Hospital, including psychiatric intensive care unit
   - development of computerised information base and service register for day-to-day and research use
   - research and planning for alcohol treatment services.

THE DISABILITY GAP

In practical terms, the intention of many of the
more recently developed parts of the service, is to
help bridge what we might call a 'disability gap'.
We can think of this in terms of a person having a
certain inherent ability to cope with life when
well. When someone becomes ill and is recovering
from illness this coping ability is almost
inevitably reduced to a greater or lesser extent.
Frequently this reduction is a temporary phenomenon,
but there can be a lengthy recuperative period which
can affect the capacity to cope in quite severe
ways, both at home, with family and friends, and at
work. In some instances some disability remains.
    Disabilities arise in three ways: firstly,
because of inherent inadequacies in personality and
upbringing. They might arise because of low
intelligence, they might arise, perhaps, as a result
of being brought up in an institution. There are
many circumstances of upbringing which result in
someone's not having had the chance to acquire the
coping ability and skills necessary for homemaking
and for putting together a way of life, especially
in a stressed, inner city environment. Secondly,
disabilities can be a result of the illness itself,
and thirdly they can result from treatment processes
themselves.
    The 'disability gap' is the difference between
the coping ability somebody demonstrates, at any
given time, and what they would expect to achieve
when well. This gap can be reduced in a number of
ways: medical services can reduce the disability
that is caused by the actual illness, but in doing
this, will also create other kinds of disabilities,
as a result of drugs, as a result of admitting a
patient to hospital, or simply as a result of
somebody becoming an outpatient and acquiring a
label. Paramedical and social services can improve
practical and social skills and provide varied
professional support. But there is rarely any
effective agency for effecting a comprehensive
programme for re-integrating someone into their own
personal social network of family, relatives,
friends and acquaintances, so that they can
relinquish the idea of being 'ill'. Having a
satisfying personal network is usually a crucial
factor in being able to accept and benefit from
medical treatment, standard social work services and
the rehousing opportunities available through the
local authority.

Our programme has been aimed at discovering
ways of making use of available resources, changing
attitudes and practices, in order to try to reduce
the non-medical part of the disability gap so that
patients can eventually make use of the available
statutory services.

PRECONDITIONS FOR CHANGE

Preconditions that we identified enabled us to set
up a network which acts at the various interfaces
and can smooth out the pattern. All the changes
noted above have been in response to - or, more
latterly, in anticipation of - perceived needs by
the community and are in no way radical or
controversial, and take maximum advantage of the
circumstances, the preconditions.

1. Serious and identifiable problems - of a
   soluble nature.
2. 'Risk-taking' environment - nothing to lose?
3. Atmosphere of collaboration rather than
   competition.
4. Willingness and ability to make flexible use of
   funds.
5. Willingness to be guided by common sense rather
   than precedent.

Obviously it is very important that problems
can be identified. All too often the problems are
quite nebulous; people know that there is something
wrong but find it difficult to pin down exactly what
it is and where the particular irritant to the
system starts. It is not easy to identify the
interface that is causing the problems, nor to be
precise about the group of clients for whome help is
needed. In Hackney we had the advantages of a 'Good
Practices' study (the first), several research
studies done in the 1970s by the Psychiatric
Rehabilitation Association (one of which was updated
in collaboration with CPRU in 1981), and our own
study, in 1979, of long-term patients.
The 'risk-taking' environment is important. One
of the difficulties with professional training is
that it does perhaps reduce the capacity to take
risks. Doctors and nurses especially have a great
deal to lose; they cannot afford to take too many
risks. One would not necessarily suggest that they
did, but they might surround themselves with a few
people who can undertake innovations and experiment
on their behalf. They can then give guidance and

perhaps act as boundary setters. This is where the
multidisciplinary nature, independent funding and
indeterminate status of CPRU is invaluable. In
Hackney we also have the benefit of a council which
is well noted for feeling that there is nothing to
lose from trying new schemes provided they are
responsibly managed.

The atmosphere of collaboration rather than
competition is difficult to engender, especially
when resources are scarce, perhaps jobs are at risk,
and, in the realms of politics, votes also. It is
worth making active efforts to reduce the scope for
conflict by agreeing priorities, sticking to
agreements and avoiding 'poaching'. It also helps
for different professions to meet informally and
learn to respect each others priorities and
abilities. How many consultant psychiatrists are on
first-name terms with social services or housing
management staff?

Funds are not always to be found from the most
obvious sources and sometimes it is necessary to
create agencies specifically to comply with the
conditions surrounding particular grants. To some
extent we have had an easy start, both in having
generous grants from the Gatsby Trust, who
recognised that money to pay for a 'secretariat' to
co-ordinate and stimulate plans was at least as
important as money for direct project work. We have
been able to use our grant very flexibly in ways
which have allowed us to make the most of offers –
of the block of flats mentioned by Adrian Lovett
(see Chapter 8) for instance – which have come our
way. We are able to redirect funds quickly and
without fuss; we are also able to use money from our
grant for capital work which will, in due course, be
repaid from income or from grants from other
sources. The Vanguard Commune houses are examples of
how this flexibility is beneficial.

PRINCIPLES

Our original programme was, in many ways, naive and
simplistic. Over the last few years we have refined
many details, but the original concepts remain
pretty well intact. Some of the principles, which
derive from the ideas discussed above, we have only
recently managed to express clearly, even though
intuition and common sense enabled them to be
incorporated early on in practice. For planning
purposes there are two essential questions: what is
needed, and how should it be provided?

1. What does each person need?
A checklist:
- accommodation
- a partner/intimate friend
- a circle of friends
- a wider network of acquaintances
- finance
- occupation during 'working' hours
- occupation during leisure time

    Answers to this question can be very simple and crude initially, for the purpose of making a start to satisfactory provisions, or can involve sophisticated assessments and formal research, discussion of which is outside the scope of this chapter.

2. How can help be given to assist each person to acquire whatever he/she cannot personally supply (see earlier discussion on disability gap)? In relation to this question we suggest the following principles as guidelines:

1. Ensure that schemes are 'real-life', rather than research constructs.
   Research should aim to serve the patients and not inhibit any chance of progress. Schemes should be planned to have permanent benefits rather than being simply for the duration of a research study.
2. Aim to make use of existing premises, facilities and staff rather than creating special (i.e. divisive) services.
   Many special projects are, on close examination, devised more for the convenience of the organisers than that of the consumers. Sheltered workshops, industrial enclave schemes, special hostels and homes may be unnecessarily divisive for some clients and will reinforce the 'disabled' or 'ill' status, making full recovery and re-integration more difficult.
3. Divide infrastructure and fixed capital resources from service agents for greater flexibility of allocation and use.
   Following the principle above, support, both with occupational stresses and in everyday life, can often be supplied independently of an actual building. A peripatetic, multi-disciplinary team can give intensive or occasional support and practical help as

required by each individual in 'ordinary' accommodation or place of work, rather than having each scheme or project separately staffed and managed. This method of providing care bears on the next principle, and obviates the necessity for a proliferation of management committees, by using existing skills and personnel in housing departments, housing associations or employers.

4. Avoid unnecessary bureaucracy and fixed capital investment.

5. Reduce 'travelling' from element to element by patient/client with the service adapting to the client's needs rather than vice versa. Continuity for the client/consumer should be stressed.

   This principle avoids both the paradox of 'punishing' a patient (for instance by requiring him to move home) for making progress, and also the disruption to progress which may occur in the course of moving from one element of a service to the other, whereby valuable time and effort is used in repairing the trauma caused by the transfer. Multidisciplinary teams and good co-ordination, especially of methods of working and ethos, between the different caring agencies, hospital and community, with overlap of personnel where possible, will mean that the difficulties which often arise at the interfaces are experienced and handled by professionals rather than by the patient.

6. Arrange services to follow a hierarchy of psychological needs, aiming to anticipate difficulties and concentrate on prevention rather than intervention in the event of a crisis.

   Experience in Hackney, and doubtless elsewhere, has shown the pointlessness of trying to provide for sophisticated needs before the simpler, basic ones have been met adequately. Patients are unlikely to take advantage of an activity designed to improve their self-esteem or social life unless their needs for a home, food and personal security are met satisfactorily.

CONCLUSIONS

In City and Hackney Health District we have taken advantage of the circumstances and preconditions

cited   above   and   have,   as   a   result,   achieved the
basic   elements   and   attitudes   for a comprehensive,
community-oriented   psychiatric   service.   The   fact
that   there   are   no   beds set aside for 'long-stay'
purposes ensures that   all   patients   live   'in   the
community' rather than in hospital. We feel that the
conscious acceptance of this method of care and   the
development   of facilities and services ancillary to
those provided by the hospital go a long way towards
raising   the   quality   of life of many patients. The
progress we have made - in a very gentle way   -   has
served   to   reduce reliance on the hospital beds and
staff and to alleviate the non-medical part   of   the
disability gap for a number of people, many of whom,
in other districts,   would   have   fallen   into   that
problematic group, the 'new' long-stay.

PART THREE

THE ELEMENTS PUT INTO PRACTICE

This section contains chapters which report on some
of the schemes which have been started as part of
comprehensive local services, in the light of general consideration of what should be incorporated
into such services and what constitutes 'good
practice'.

Dr Donald Dick, in his main chapter, presents
an imaginative outline of what services should be
'captured' and set up in each district. His visits
to many services throughout the country in his years
as Director of the Health Advisory Service give him
a unique perspective and it is notable that he,
along with many others, places considerable emphasis
on co-ordination, good organisation and personal
factors in securing an effective service.

In her discussion, Mrs Edith Morgan uses her
own considerable experience of the birth and growth
of mental health projects all over the country to
enlarge on many aspects, with particular attention
paid to ways in which the voluntary movement can
contribute to a service.

Three of the seminar chapters describe specific
projects: a joint hostel scheme, a community mental
health centre and a psychogeriatric day hospital.
The other two chapters report on psychiatric issues
in general practice and an administrator's experiences of working the system on behalf of mental
illness and community services.

Chapter Fourteen

SERVICES IN THE NET

Donald H Dick

Providing a mental health service for a community is a very complex matter. It involves many people and many organisations, each with different central preoccupations and often with different objectives. The complexity begins with even superficial thought about definitions of what constitutes mental health or mental ill health, and who in a community should be doing something about it. In trying to arrive at definitions, for example, it is easy to become stuck on the continuum that ranges, at one end, from the severely psychotic patient in need of treatment for a disease of the brain, to the other end, where an individual may be unhappy about imperfections in experience measured against the expectations of a high-drive consumer society preoccupied with affluence and sex. Freud got it about right when he said that health is the ability to work and to love.

And who should be responsible for the mental health of a community? No single person or organisation can possibly control all that influences a community's mental health. Apart from social attitudes, prejudices and enthusiasms, there are many self-determining organisations and services which contribute to the whole. What they contribute may be only a part of their total task and may be shared with other groups and other problems. There will be specialist psychiatric services and general health services, like general practice. There are specialist social workers and general social work teams with obligations to other groups of people, like the elderly, children, the mentally handicapped and the physically handicapped. Welfare, home care and residential services are also shared with other groups. There are services for housing, employment and education which have widespread obligations and yet which each make a vital contribution to the restoration and maintenance of the mentally ill to a normal life.

Another set of circles that touches the mentally ill are the legal and penal systems. There are individuals with mental illness before the courts, contacts with the police, the probation service, the prisons, the special hospitals, medium secure units, forensic psychiatry services. There is also the balance between treatment, liberty and security contained in mental health legislation that enters the question.

In each community there are voluntary organisations which are either branches of national bodies, such as MIND, the National Schizophrenia Fellowship, Alcoholics Anonymous, Anorexics Aid, or local and unique developments for a particular purpose. Self-help and support groups are growing rapidly in numbers throughout the western world. The consumer movement gathers strength in health as in other spheres, year by year. Beyond that we are influenced by economic, demographic and sociological changes, all of which have implications for the mentally ill and what happens to them.

In each community there is, therefore, what is known as a network of services and organisations available to the mentally ill. Sometimes the services work in partnership, sometimes separately, asking for help in times of need. Occasionally they are well co-ordinated. More often they thirst for knowledge and information about each other. Edith Morgan, Director of the Good Practices in Mental Health Project, reports that one of the advantages of asking a community to search for its own good practice in mental health is to strengthen contacts and communication and to induce serious discussion on the nature and quality of local services (see discussion following).

The aim of this chapter is to look at the sum of all these contributions, especially from the point of view of specialist mental health services, and to see what practical lessons can be drawn from the experiences of diverse communities throughout England and Wales. I want to see if we can be sure of finding that all the divisions of the army engaged in the battle are at least marching to the sound of the same gun-fire. We can start by standing back to see the whole picture in outline. Immediately, there is a snag over language and the preoccupation with what is important to different levels in the system of care. The service providers speak a language of clinical problems, problem-

solving for individuals, treatment needs and daily
pressures. The management and organisation providers
speak a language of budgets, strategy priorities and
planning. These are the landowners of the care
system and have, perforce, to use a language that
puts some meaning into expressions like national
priority services, resource allocation working party
targets, capital and manpower planning, the revenue
consequences of capital spending, performance indicators, strategic planning, operational planning,
joint planning, joint financing, growth money,
monitoring policy objectives, cost effectiveness,
cost efficiency, opportunity costing.

This is the Norman-French of the landowners,
which helps to keep the fieldworkers and peasantry
(puzzled and hard at work) excluded from making
irritating demands unless they, too, can understand
and manipulate the language for themselves. There is
nothing new in this. All professions invent their
own language and thereby corner the knowledge and
power that exclusiveness gives. The peasant just
wants peace in which to sow his beans and milk his
cow. The fieldworkers in health and social services
and the managers too, want to be allowed to get on
with the business of treating the distressed, sick
or incapable people who come their way. They want to
be protected from marauding bands of efficiency
experts, line managers, staff organisations, local
politicians and Community Health Councils with bees
in their bonnets. Nobody is too keen on busybodies
like the Health Advisory Service, the Social Work
Service, the National Development Team, the Royal
Colleges, the Bean Marketing Board who all know how
to do it better. Lest you should think I am
discriminating, the high-priests of MIND and other
national bodies are not always totally popular.

Now whilst it is fascinating to look at the
interplay between the different parts of the
organisational structure, it does not seem to be
very helpful in seeing how to make a better service
to meet the needs of the people. It is almost as if
we have stepped back to see the wood from the trees
and found ourselves in a semantic bog. I believe
that there is a better point of view.

The average health district has a population of
about 200,000 people. That is a crowd to fill
Wembley Stadium more than twice over, or a good-
sized city. If we could look down upon that crowd in
its own houses and streets, and by some means
identify different categories of people, we would
see some very interesting things. For example, there

would be about 30,000 people aged 65 or over. Ten
per cent, which is 3,000, would be showing evidence
of senile dementia. Only a minority would be in
hospital and a few more than that in residential
homes. Most would be at home, and around them would
be clustered family and friends helping to support
them. There would be 1,600 people with schizophrenia. We would all be surprised by the small
proportion in hospital, probably nearer 100 than 200
at any one time, and in some districts more like 50
or 60. The great majority would be at home and
fending for themselves with more or less success.
There would be close on 3,000 people with various
forms of severe depressive illness or manic
depressive illness, not all ill at once, but with a
need for treatment at times. There would be somewhat
above 1,500 people with drinking problems severe
enough to be called alcoholism, and many more not
far off it. Around those would be grouped three or
four times that number of family members affected by
the alcohol abuse of the drinking member. Twenty-
five people in any one year would commit suicide.
About ten times that number would attempt it. There
would be children and young people in distress,
behaviourally disturbed, making their way towards
mental illness or borstals. There would be those in
contact with both health services and the legal
system, some in secure units, some in prison, some
under supervision. There might be a group of 30 or
so who are addicted to drugs. There would, of
course, be lots of people who are unemployed,
unhappy or lonely, or not very capable or
excessively anxious or troubled by their marriages
or their sex lives, who from time to time need help
from general practitioners, social workers,
counsellors and others prepared to help.
Occasionally, they would need specialist psychiatric
care. Then there are the homeless, the unemployable
and those who drift through the streets, to the doss
house, the railway arches and eventually the
mortuary.
     But the majority of citizens go busily about
their business, able to work and love and play
without much thought for those around them who can
do none of these things. Until, that is, they are
personally involved. If the same all-seeing eye
could identify the citizens who earn their living in
the mental health professions, we would again be
surprised by what we saw. Almost everyone would be
found within the walls of the buildings of the
psychiatric service. We would be forgiven for

thinking that the few that we saw out and about
beyond the walls were missionaries sent out into a
hostile environment. About 95 per cent of all
psychiatrically-trained staff are to be found
working inside hospitals, and only five per cent
outside, including day hospitals. Almost exactly the
opposite is true of the people identified as
mentally ill: five per cent in hospital, 95 per cent
in their own homes or domestic accommodation. Other
people working with the mentally ill or distressed
in the community would be seen sometimes in their
buildings, sometimes in the homes of their patients.
After a time it would become apparent that groups
form networks amongst themselves, now working with
staff in hospitals, now with social work teams, now
with the housing department, now within voluntary
organisations. There would be pathways between
different buildings; County Hall, the health
authority, the planners' department, the head-
quarters of voluntary organisations.

One feature might become apparent. There would
be some mentally ill people who would find no place
to rest or receive help, some for whom there was no
suitable service. There would be others who cannot
leave the place where they have been sent for want
of anywhere else to go: the persistent, unrepentant
drunk, the aggressive, antisocial person, perhaps
the disturbed adolescent, even the incontinent,
confused old lady.

This view of how a community is meeting the
needs of its mentally ill members gives rise to one
very obvious question. How should all the
contributions be organised into a comprehensive
service? For if they are not organised, there is
likely to be a duplication of some services, over-
provision of others and gaps for which no one has
taken responsibility. The effectiveness may go
unexamined and a lot of money may be spent without
balance between competing demands. Even in the
Cinderella services, there are some that are more
popular than others, which must be protected. There
are plenty of district services that are doing
excellent work in some respects, even earning the
title of 'centre of excellence' for a particular
specialised department, and yet who do not even know
that they have serious gaps in what they offer by
way of comprehensive care.

How is comprehensiveness to be achieved? How is
the balance of even development to be maintained? I
propose to describe some practical systems that are
to be seen around the country which appear capable

of solving some of the problems of co-ordination and
the delivery of a comprehensive service. First I
shall tell you why I do not think that the present
system of planning and management of service
delivery is working. In the reorganised and
restructured health service, it is supposed that a
small group of health and social services staff, the
joint health care planning team, can by themselves
come up with plans for mental health that will serve
the needs of the community. This group, a rep-
resentative selection of the best informed professionals, is expected to write out a shopping list
of what they believe to be needed. The specialist
plan is taken by the District Team of Officers or
the Social Services Management Team or their joint
officer group, the Joint Care Planning Team, put
into some sort of priority order and then presented
to the health authority, the Social Services
Committee or the Joint Consultative Committee to be
adopted and declared as authority policy,
implemented or not according to the money available
for growth in the following year. The main product
of this industry is paper and the by-product is
frustration. The shopping list has been written
before the menu has been decided upon. Some of the
dishes cannot be cooked for lack of the right
ingredients – and no one brought the money anyway.
Development is surely a cycle:

- Need is recognised;
- Someone has a vision of what will meet the
  need;
- A strategy is prepared on the steps to be taken
  to reach the vision;
- A decision is taken on the order of steps to be
  followed;
- Resources are found;
- Detailed plans are made;
- They are implemented;
- The outcome is evaluated against the original
  need.

The cycle turns, finding better ways of meeting the
needs or throwing up new ones which now stand
revealed.
    Translated into the development of mental
health services, this view requires a succession of
special groups to make a contribution and pass it on
to the next phase. The first phase, perceiving the
need, is a job for the whole community. It is the
sum of the complaints, the missing services, the

exclusions, the observations of the professional staff who recognise gaps, the observations of the Community Health Council and voluntary organisations, the shortfalls measured against regional or national norms, and understanding of morbidity and the pressure of publicity and scandal. Two elements are needed in this phase:

1. A good information system;
2. Some form of community mental health interest group.

Good information about morbidity and present performance is primarily the responsibility of the community physician and his department and in detail the mental health service. The best services seem to be strong on information. The practical manifestations are regular performance statistics, an annual report and analysis of trends.

Mental health interest groups have played a very important part in some districts in generating widespread interest and debate. Some of them have been a happy consequence of a Good Practices in Mental Health (GPMH) project. If anyone at all can contribute, there needs to be no argument about how all the interested parties put in their pennyworth. I believe it is a wise district that puts money into servicing such a group, allowing thinking time, creating a forum in which ideas can ferment.

Next, a strategy must be generated. Finding a vision to meet particular needs is a task for small groups with specialist knowledge. In mental health services a single group cannot comfortably cover the whole range. There are a number of distinct areas of interest which each need their champions: acute psychiatry; psychiatry of chronic mental illness, including rehabilitation; psychiatry of old age; psychiatry of alcohol abuse; psychiatry of drug abuse; psychiatry of childhood and adolescence; forensic psychiatry and the psychiatry of disruptive behaviour. Running across these functions are the ways of combining work like community psychiatry, sector teamwork or specialist departments with a research interest. Each of these, to my mind, deserves the attention of a group of people who are given the work of developing the community's response to the perceived needs. This is not to suggest a proliferation of committees. It is to make sure that natural working groups know that one of their tasks is development, that if they do not do it, no one else will and there is no point in trying to find someone else to blame if nothing is happening. All the work of health and social

services is done in small groups, each with
different functions. It is better if the understanding of the purpose of each is conscious. In
many districts there are groups identified by a name
with a definite project in mind: the Department of
Mental Health for the Elderly or the CPRU, for
example. My conclusion is that such a group of local
champions is essential as a link between the needs
of the mentally ill and the decisions to be made
about the use of resources.

The next phase belongs to the officers of the
various authorities, the District Management Team or
social services management group. They have
territorial responsibility and must put into some
order of priority the competing requests from many
sources. They can also take advice on some of the
wilder suggestions. The outcome is a presentation of
suggested policies with indications of priority to
the responsible authority, the district health
authority, the social services committee or their
Joint Consultative Committee. The outcome should be
a strategic plan or joint strategic plan for mental
illness services which is really a set of policy
objectives with agreement to commit resources in a
certain order of priority.

Although all the steps are important, the next
step is essential. Without it, all the effort so far
is pointless and all that follows is fruitless.
Money has to be found. It is not enough to rely on
growth money which is now negligible. It is no good
being bitter about not having enough central funds.
If money is to be found in addition to slow growth,
it has to come from the deployment of existing
resources, known as opportunity costing. What
sacrifices have to be made in one area, to make
gains in another? There is some hard bargaining to
be done. You have only to think of the fury that is
roused when it is proposed to close a much-loved but
surplus and expensive local community hospital.
Money does not easily pass from a nursing budget
into an occupational therapy budget, nor from health
services to social services. The capital and revenue
of mental health services are locked up in large
institutions. Freeing them is a long and tedious
process but it can be successfully planned. In the
next decade the site of care of the mentally ill
will inevitably change from institutional to
domestic. A number of initiatives have already
begun. Programmes of steady transfer are beginning,
following the broad principles of the Worcester
Project. Some major hospitals are already planning

the details of condensation and eventual closure. If
resources are freed for development, detailed
planning can begin. This is followed by
implementation and delivery of the improved service
to the community.

There is, of course, a final stage: the
evaluation of the outcome. Has the achievement of
policy objectives met the need which they were
designed to meet? We are back round the cycle to a
good information system and the examination of
whether the needs of the community are being met.

Key staff in a comprehensive mental health
service have a number of roles and may belong to
several of the small groups described. In their
different disciplines they may be the master
craftsman of their own professional skills, the
planner, the advocate, the adviser, the manager, the
innovator but sometimes the brickwall, the
obstructor hoarding his possessions and defending
his territory, preventing others from making
progress.

The feature of a good service that excites me
most when visiting is not the excellence of
buildings, not the generous staff establishment, not
the superb paperwork or organisation charts but the
spirit of the highly effective group at work: the
group that believes itself to be uniquely blessed in
the compatibility of its members who can together
reach the sky. The group that knows its task and
combines both the health of the group as a whole and
the needs of individual members.

If the groups making up the service are in good
group health and if their links with other groups
are sound, they will create the network of services
that we are looking for. Conscious attention paid to
the way that groups function, both individually and
as a whole, will take a community's mental health
service a long way towards improved performance.
Those that identify themselves as responsible for
that performance should therefore nurture group
effectiveness with especial care. Have you noticed
the growing adoption by Western industry of the
Japanese concept of quality circles? Circles of
workers at all levels are asked to make self-
appraisal of the effectiveness and efficiency of
their performance and suggest remedies. It is widely
held that it is because of techniques like this that
Japan out-performs its competitors.

This paper has addressed a complex problem. I
hope that some themes have emerged that will be of
value in approaching it. Clearly we live in

interesting times in mental health. But, as the
Chinese say, that is not necessarily a blessing.

DISCUSSION AND COMMENTS

Edith Morgan

The description that Dr Dick gives of what is likely
to be happening, in mental health terms, to the
people living in any one health district is most
illuminating. It makes bald statistics a good deal
more intelligible though not, perhaps, more
palatable. As he spoke I found myself adding to the
numbers he gave the numbers of others - families,
friends, neighbours and workmates - also affected.
What one then sees are communities which are often
very troubled. It was startling, too, to be reminded
that 95 per cent of all psychiatrically trained
staff are employed inside hospitals, while the same
proportion of people who have been diagnosed as
mentally ill are, in fact, outside those hospitals.
His references to lack of co-operation between
official bodies, especially between health and
social services has a drearily familiar ring. Lord
Trefgarne emphasised that co-operation and
collaboration will make or break community-based
psychiatric services, and Dr Dick goes further by
proposing down-to-earth ways for overcoming the
separation of responsibility for planning and
management. The flexibility and informality of the
arrangements he suggests for mental health interest
groups, natural specialist working groups and local
champions are attractive, involving, as they do,
whole communities rather than a selected few. At the
same time, there must be some anxiety about how to
make sure that the findings of such groups are
actually heeded.
    I have particular sympathy with the points made
by all speakers about money not being the answer to
all problems. Of course, no responsible person would
say that money does not matter, but some of the
other resources that are needed to produce change
and improvement are just as important.
    The World Health Organisation made a study of
constraints in developing mental health services in
1977. In their report they said that before the

working party met the members expected to be told
that the greatest constraints in each of the
countries studied stemmed from limitations of money
and other resources. But that was not what they
found. They concluded that the biggest obstacles to
progress were such things as apathy, inertia and
lack of flexibility. The WHO working party
identified information as an essential key to
progress. This finding has been borne out in many of
the chapters in this book. It was dissatisfaction
with the sparseness of information about mental
health services which are functioning satisfactorily
which led us, also in 1977, to set up the Good
Practices in Mental Health Project. The GPMH
Information Service (see bibliography) that has
grown out of the project is being well used,
confirming that people concerned with mental health
do need, and want to share, knowledge and
experience.

What else should go into Dr Dick's net? We are
fortunate in this country to have a voluntary
movement that already contributes a great deal to
mental health - more than is generally realised. It
can contribute still more, though not necessarily in
the ways some people would select. Currently,
volunteers and voluntary bodies are exceedingly
popular - to an extent that can, at times, be
worrying since some professionals see them as a
means of unloading work and responsibilities that
they find too difficult. When they succeed in doing
this it can lead to disaster and disillusionment for
everyone involved. Most of all, it harms those for
whom the help was being organised in the first
place.

Misuse by some professionals is only part of
the story, and a remarkable feature of the voluntary
movement is the number of people working
professionally in mental health who spend their
spare time as volunteers. As well as adding to the
weight of general activity they help a great deal by
feeding in knowledge, and can build up much needed
confidence amongst non-professional volunteers to
use their own particular skills and abilities. It is
exeedingly important that professional volunteers
refrain from dominating their organisation and from
stifling initiative or criticism.

The membership of voluntary mental health
associations also includes a large proportion of
people who have had personal experience of mental
illness, either through being ill themselves or
having a close relative who is ill. It is still

difficult for people to declare openly that they are
one of the group labelled 'mentally ill', and
perhaps this is why the self-help movement is not as
strong in mental health as in some other health and
social problem areas. What this means, in effect, it
that there is a vast amount of information within
voluntary organisations from the point of view of
people who use the mental health services. The
experience and wishes of consumers are at present
not taken sufficiently into account in the planning
and management of these services, and there is an
urgent need to find ways of reaching directly the
people who have the greatest interest of anyone in
improving mental health care.

Dr Dick touched on the tricky problems of co-
operation between professionals and volunteers. This
is indeed an important issue, not only in this
country but internationally. A seminar held in 1982
identified some of the 'hot spots' and also set out
some of the principles conducive to effective
collaboration (Gordon 1982). To say that the basis
is mutual respect and understanding is, perhaps,
platitudinous; it is nevertheless true.

An underlying theme of this book is how to
bring about change, and every time this is discussed
it seems more difficult to achieve. Yet change does
happen. Looking back to my first student visit to a
mental hospital, 30 years ago, and on my 20 years
with MIND, I find it incredible how much change was
taking place, almost imperceptibly, throughout these
years. Some of the change was a result of national
campaigns, legislation and directives. But much more
of it was started at a local level by individuals or
small groups. Somebody had an idea and had the
energy to find the resources to try it out. If it
worked it was taken up by others and sometimes
became widespread. Two of those early ideas, which I
saw from the beginning, are now normal mental health
service practice. One was the scheme introduced by
Dr T P Rees at Warlingham Park Hospital, for nurses
to follow-up patients in the community - the
forerunner of the highly valued community
psychiatric nursing service. The other example was a
group home, set up in 1962 by the local mental
health association in Ealing. One of these examples
was a professional innovation, the other voluntary.
The common factor is that both were <u>local</u> in origin.
Dr Dick has emphasised the vital importance of local
planning, and perhaps even a district of 200,000
should be sub-divided for some aspects of planning
and delivery of service. I am very much in favour of

the patchwork approach.
     It was this kind of experience, repeated many
times during my years in developing MIND's community
programme, that led me to set up the Good Practices
in Mental Health Project in the way I did. I have
learned a great deal from the GPMH project:

- that with the exception of a few diehards
  people can be encouraged to work co-operatively
  with other groups, especially when their
  interests are not threatened and the work is as
  positive as a GPMH study;
- that local groups are deeply concerned about
  preventing mental ill-health. They select for
  inclusion in a study, over and over again,
  community schemes which are supporting people
  at crisis points or through periods of
  particular stress;
- that voluntary bodies and individual
  volunteers, far from being know-all busybodies,
  are over-modest about the contribution they
  make;
- that there is a thirst for information, not
  only about what fellow practitioners are doing
  300 miles away, but also about what is
  happening just down the road.

     Finally, a word about the pace at which we
should be pressing for change - or trying to
transfer services into Dr Dick's community net.
There are those who would like to see a community
psychiatric service, accompanied by closure of all
the large mental hospitals, practically overnight,
and by decree. As many of you will know, this is
what took place in Italy in 1978. In most places
community services were inadequate or non-existent,
and the resulting chaos was disastrous. There is a
lesson in this, though we are, perhaps, well enough
protected by our cautious British character. At the
same time we have to guard against those who say
that the introduction of community psychiatric
services must wait until the 'community' is ready
for it. Certainly it is true that attempts to impose
unreasonable burdens will create a backlash;
undoubtedly communities and professionals alike will
resist any proposal to send large numbers of
patients out from closing hospitals without proper
preparation and support. But community acceptance of
rational schemes can be accomplished. The last item,
therefore, that I would place in Dr Dick's net is a
comprehensive, well-planned programme of education,

based   not   upon   manipulating public opinion but on
honest   facts and information and a modicum of faith
in shared humanity.

REFERENCE

Gordon P (ed) (1982). Professionals and   Volunteers:
   Partners   or Rivals? Report of a seminar organised
   by The World Federation for   Mental   Health.   King
   Edward's Hospital Fund for London.

Chapter Fifteen

REHABILITATION AND COMMUNITY CARE: WORKING TOGETHER

Mark A J O'Callaghan

INTRODUCTION

Once again we are urged to make efforts to provide more community care in the mental health field. The government has shown its commitment by putting out various documents in which health and social services are encouraged to co-operate in helping to shift the balance of psychiatric care towards the community; it has helped more recently by extending the joint financing arrangements (DHSS 1983).

Whilst there are guidelines as to how to use the money (and upon what to spend it) in order to achieve greater community psychiatric care, there is little in the way of advice in the most difficult area, that of promoting good working relationships on the ground. Indeed, it could be argued that it is not so much the lack of money that prevents greater co-operation in the mental health field towards providing a comprehensive service, but rather the will and especially the methods to do so.

This chapter describes how the health service and local authority have co-operated with voluntary agencies in setting up facilities in Solihull which attempt to achieve the aim of providing a comprehensive community-based psychiatric service. Following a brief explanation of how joint financing money was used to set up the scheme, we outline the obstacles which hinder close co-operation, and then suggest how they might be overcome. The evaluation of the joint system is then discussed, together with difficulties and the steps taken to remedy them. Finally, we describe some plans for the future. In reporting our work I am writing on behalf also of my colleagues, Kunal Raychaudhuri, Peter Davidson, Trevor O'Neil, Patrick Wallace, and Colin Grierson.

BACKGROUND TO THE ESTABLISHMENT OF THE JOINT SYSTEM

Like many other psychiatric hospitals, Hollymoor
Hospital in south Birmingham has witnessed a decline
in bed numbers (over 40 per cent) since the 1950s.
The reduction of the long-stay population was
considerably helped by the establishment of the
Rehabilitation Unit in 1972 by Kunal Raychaudhuri,
consultant psychiatrist. Following **Better Services
for the Mentally Ill** (DHSS 1975) discussion took
place between health and social services planners,
mainly through the Care Planning Team (Mentally
Ill), for the establishment of Middlewood House as a
community rehabilitation hostel and day centre to
provide a service working jointly with, and
complementing, that of the hospital. The scheme,
piloted by Peter Davidson, (Assistant Director,
Solihull Social Services) came to fruition with the
completion of a building costing £470,000. £115,000
of this was contributed by the health authority
under joint financing arrangements. Running costs
are shared on a seven-year tapering formula with 60
per cent of the first year's (1980-1981) costs being
met by the health authority. Middlewood House took
its first clients in April 1980.
   The first major difficulty that we faced in our
attempts to work towards a comprehensive mental
health service is that while the boundaries of
Solihull Metropolitan Borough Social Services
Department and Solihull Health District are
coterminous, their mental health catchment areas are
not. The northern part of Solihull Borough is served
by Highcroft Psychiatric Hospital (administered by
North Birmingham Health District), the south by
Central Hospital (South Warwickshire Health
District), and the centre by Hollymoor Hospital
(under Solihull Health District). In addition,
Hollymoor Hospital provides psychiatric cover to
parts of central and east Birmingham; it lies some
ten miles from the nearest part of its catchment
area. Middlewood House is situated in Chelmsley
Wood, in the northern part of Solihull and therefore
in Highcroft Hospital's catchment area. Attempts at
co-operation must take these factors into account.

PRINCIPLES OF REHABILITATION AND COMMUNITY CARE

An important aspect of any joint rehabilitation and
community care approach is that facilities should be
complementary and part of an overall framework. I
was appointed in late 1979, as clinical

psychologist, to help reorganise the hospital rehabilitation unit as well as to set up Middlewood House; this post is also joint financed. Similar policy documents were drawn up for both units based upon five main principles.

The first principle is that people should be encouraged to be as independent and as community-based as possible. A survey carried out in the 1950s revealed that many admissions to Hollymoor Hospital had a large social component. A more recent survey revealed similar findings. Our aim now is to see whether some of these people might be more appropriately placed in Middlewood House rather than going to a hospital admission ward. Of course, they may still need psychiatric help, but this can be provided on an outpatient basis if necessary. Even admission to Middlewood House is considered carefully so that someone with family problems, for example, may be offered help at home rather than being admitted to our residential provision. Clearly, such a system relies heavily on each element having the support of the next along the continuum of provision. The community-based support services have the backing of Middlewood House which in turn needs the support of the hospital rehabilitation unit.

The second, and related, principle is that training should take place in the appropriate place and with appropriate provisions. We must again be guided by the aim of complementarity. We should provide a range of facilities so that patients on long-stay wards have opportunities to take the first steps towards independence without being seriously (and detrimentally) disoriented. We should also provide appropriate training accommodation for those about to leave hospital.

To provide training kitchens wards have been converted to have appropriate cooking facilities (gas and electric). This need not be an expensive proposition in all cases, and sometimes capital expenditure can lead to savings in running costs, such as occurred at Middlewood House. The conversion of the main 'institutionalised' kitchen into three training kitchen units (two gas, one electric) within the one room (so that they could be supervised by the domestic supervisor) cost about £2,000 (joint finance money). It knocked around £5,000 off the catering budget within a year as well as promoting greater independence of the clients in working towards self-catering.

The next principle is that appropriate training

strategies should be used rather than some of the
'technology-based' techniques of training currently
in use elsewhere. Thus, for example, we felt that
instead of training clients to get tokens for
emitting 'appropriate' eye-contact in artificial
social skills training sessions (after training the
staff how to give the tokens appropriately!) and
then weaning them off the technology-based token
economy system, we should train them how to make
friends irrespective of poor eye-contact at times.

A related principle is that the natural (or
real-life) consequences of a person's behaviour
should influence our rehabilitees' actions as far as
possible. We believe that with proper training this
encourages a person to take responsibility for
his/her own actions. When a patient on a
rehabilitation ward deliberately broke some windows
there, he was charged with the offence by the
police, taken to court and fined by the magistrates
who recognised that merely by being in a psychiatric
hospital with a psychiatric diagnosis did not mean
that he could not be held responsible for his own
actions.

OBSTACLES TO CO-OPERATION

Although necessary, the establishment of community
facilities alongside existing health service
provision, as well as the development of policies
based upon the principles outlines above, were not
sufficient prerequisites for co-operation. The very
establishment of a facility like Middlewood House
leads to difficulties. Hospital staff may view it as
a threat to them in two ways. Firstly, because it
appears in line with the government's declared
intention to transfer the burden of psychiatric care
towards the community and concomittently some
resources as well. Middlewood House may be seen as a
first step along the road to achieving this aim,
therefore heralding the draining of already scarce
resources from the hospital. Secondly, Middlewood
House may be seen as a threat to the professional
integrity of members of the nursing and allied
discipline in the hospital. The argument runs that
if the (generally poorly-trained) residential social
work staff can be successful in rehabilitating
psychiatric patients then this may cast doubt upon
the professional abilities of hospital staff. Thus,
success at Middlewood House may be seen as being
bought at the expense of hospital staff.

Care has also to be taken to ensure that

Middlewood House does not replicate the work of the
rehabilitation unit at Hollymoor Hospital so that
other provision is lacking. The services provided
should be complementary; both must agree on the type
of client and stage of training suited to each
facility.

Two catchwords describe the poor relationship
which is often found between hospitals and social
services facilities: 'dumping' and 'creaming'. With
regard to the first, social services hostels are
frightened that the hosptal will 'dump' their worst
patients (in terms of problem behaviour and/or
chronicity). From the hospital side, staff are
concerned that the hostel will 'cream' off the easy
cases and get the credit for quick successes,
leaving the hospital to cope with the more
intractable patients. This situation is worsened for
referrals from the community or some other agency
for clients who exhibit problem behaviour. In such
cases the client may be shuttled between hospital
and hostel with the hospital saying that the case is
one which more properly belongs to the social
services and the hostel saying that the hospital
should be involved instead. The client in the middle
inevitably suffers.

PRACTICAL ASPECTS OF CO-OPERATION

In order to overcome the problems outlined above a
number of measures were taken. An important first
step was the appointment of a clinical psychologist
(myself) to work at both places. This had a number
of major effects. Firstly, by working at both places
I could ensure that duplication of work was
minimized. Secondly, I could help to set criteria
for the type of rehabilitee each place could help.
Thirdly, my being involved at both units lessened
the likelihood of 'dumping' and 'creaming' taking
place. I was aware of the backgrounds of the
candidates who were being put forward by the
hospital as being suitable for the hostel. If the
hostel refused to take a client I would have to help
justify that decision to colleagues at the hospital.
Fourthly, I could act as a purveyor of information
between the units, and, more importantly, act as an
'honest broker' between them in cases of difficult
or 'borderline' referrals. A psychologist is useful
in this respect in having no traditional ties with
either the nursing or medical professions on the one
hand, or social workers on the other. He is
therefore less likely to be seen as being biased

towards either the hospital or the hostel. Finally, I have been able to provide an evaluation of the whole service.

The second important step was the decision to make communication as easy as possible to prevent mutual suspicions accumulating. At the regular weekly meetings at the rehabilitation unit a member of Middlewood staff is present and hospital staff attend Middlewood meetings. Members of staff take it in turn to be present at meetings so that they all become involved in the exchange of information.

The third step was to establish common language and practices. At first we had separate initial application and assessment forms. Gradually we worked towards closer integration so that now we have common forms at both establishments. These forms are now also used at a voluntary rehabilitation hostel run by Birmingham Association for Mental Health (MIND) who wished to co-operate with us. A related step was the carrying out of joint assessments on occasion. For instance, joint assessment was helpful for a woman detained at Rampton Hospital. In conjunction with the local interim secure unit, we worked out a programme of rehabilitation so that she would pass through all our units in a planned fashion. As well as carrying out joint assessments we also conduct joint reviews of progress.

Although Middlewood House advertises that it is not a medical centre, nevertheless it appreciates the need for support from Hollymoor Hospital, without which it would lack the security to help difficult clients. Middlewood has been far more likely to take such patients from the hospital because of this support. If, at the end of the month's trial, Middlewood House is deemed inappropriate for the client then the hospital will take the responsibility for readmitting or finding alternative accommodation.

An important issue in trying to get closer working co-operation between two facilities is that each should be aware of what the other is doing on the day-to-day level. We started off a pilot scheme with the officer-in-charge at Middlewood House, Patrick Wallace, working on the main rehabilitation ward at Hollymoor and then the charge nurse on that ward, Trevor O'Neil, spending an equal amount of time at Middlewood House. We now have regular interchange of staff, so that those who are working 'on the ground' get to know what their colleagues are doing, can get experience of good practices

which they can introduce in their own setting, and
easily discuss anything which they feel might not be
in a client's best interests.

A similar useful exercise is joint visits to
other units. It is helpful to go as a combined
multidisciplinary team from both units and visit a
whole system so that proper evaluation and
discussion can take place in the light of our own
work. As a Joint National Demonstration Centre
others visit us in a similar fashion. We ask that a
multidisciplinary team visits us rather than a
couple of individuals from the same profession, and
we suggest that as well as learning from us we wish
to learn and benefit from the experience of our
visitors.

We are now in the process of setting up joint
training and education with other agencies including
the Department of Extramural Studies at Birmingham
University. The sharing of resources and expertise
for training with other rehabilitation systems means
that it can be carried out more economically. We are
now trying to provide training in a workshop format
which can be video-taped and kept for reference and
use by new members of staff.

Finally, we arrange occasional socials to which
we invite other local agencies. A small group of
people from Hollymoor Rehabilitation Unit,
Middlewood House and Birmingham Association of
Mental Health Rehabilitation Hostel, Charles Davis
House, meet for a meal each month. The importance of
such informal contacts cannot be underestimated
since they generate a lot of goodwill and practical
discussion.

EVALUATION OF THE JOINT SYSTEM

One of the more important aspects of our work is to
monitor the service. Every six months I, as the
psychologist, provide a report based upon statistics
and comments supplied by members of both units. The
aim of this report is not just to provide a static
evaluation of our work in terms of overall success
or failure but to provide dynamic picture of
strengths and weakness in order that we might
develop our system further. The statistics that we
collect in the main come from within the system with
no special data-gathering exercises.

Although we obtain data about readmission,
symptom frequency and severity, problem behaviour
and independence skills, we are more concerned that
there is an evaluation of the 'quality' of client's

life. Have we enriched it? We may have lessened a
client's 'problem behaviour' of inappropriate
seeking of attention from staff by suicidal gestures
but it may have resulted in isolation and
loneliness. We can be guided by information from the
voluntary sector. Clearly, we could appear to be
successful if we reduce our readmission rates
dramatically. However, if this is at the expense of
people almost having their hands stapled to their
front door in order to prevent readmission then we
have not done our job properly. A consumer
evaluation of our service has been invaluable,
particularly in the day centre at Middlewood where,
together with statistics of attendances and absence
rates for particular sessions, it has helped us to
plan timetables better geared to our clients' needs.
    The next section of the evaluation of our
rehabilitation system looks at families. One of our
chief concerns is that individuals should not be
seen in isolation from their family and living
situation. From an investigation of our readmissions
over three years we discovered that family or
marital disharmony was one of the main precipitating
factors in relapse. For example, failure to take
adequate account of family disharmony over money has
led to some 28 readmissions for a thirty-two year
old woman. Her pattern is one of emergency
admission, stabilisation on her medication and then
discharge home without the underlying problems ever
being tackled. A difficulty is that by trying to
shift the burden of psychiatric care into the
community we are placing it on some of the people
who are least able to cope with it, namely the
families. We have therefore attempted, through the
local branch of the National Schizophrenia
Fellowship, to survey the problems faced by
families. Help of this kind will eventually become
part of our regular work with each admission.
    Our recent work with families illustrates our
collaboration with the voluntary sector. For
instance, we were able to recommend to certain
families that they attend a course run by a
psychologist from a neighbouring hospital (Walsgrave
in Coventry) in conjunction with the Birmingham
branch of the National Schizophrenia Fellowship. At
Hollymoor we run a relatives' and landlord/ladies'
evening from time to time so that they can meet the
Rehabilitation Unit staff. At Middlewood House we
encouraged the setting up of the 'Focus Club' at
which relatives and friends meet regularly to share
problems and where they can call upon staff from our

joint system to provide advice and support. For those families needing more intensive help we have set up a pilot family therapy project using social workers from our joint system and the general hospital service. The local Community Voluntary Service has provided us with facilities to hold the sessions and a local registered charity 'ANSWER' has provided us with money to help run it.

Our next area of evaluation is staff, since not only must we evaluate the burden on families but also that placed on our staff. A consumer evaluation by staff is extremely useful. A high turnover rate of staff going to similar grades of posts elsewhere could indicate general dissatisfaction with the work they are doing, but this is complicated by the system of compulsory rotation amongst nursing staff. Sickness rates are another useful indicator of staff satisfaction and stress. Figures reveal that generally the sickness rates on both our units are lower than those which occur in similar establishments elsewhere.

The next two areas indicate how other agencies and the local community see our work. The approach here is again a consumer evaluation. We are trying to develop Middlewood as a community centre and were greatly assisted in this by a request from the local Brownie pack to use our large community room at Middlewood House. The sight of Brownies coming in every Tuesday has been a great help in showing that our residents pose no dangers for children. Research carried out by the Department of Psychology at Birmingham University showed that attitudes to Middlewood House were fairly positive and similar to those towards a local church community centre.

Finally, we are trying to evaluate our full system, looking at policies to see if they need to be changed. We have already carried out a review to discover restrictive practices within our system and to check if these are appropriate. We have found few such practices and those present tend to lessen as one moves through the system towards Middlewood House. Another review indicates how well the units are functioning and what changes might be needed. Three major developments are indicated

First of all, our two medium- to long-term rehabilitation wards are not working as well as they might. Investigation of flows through these wards revealed a fairly stagnant population; a result of inappropriate mixing of people with different needs. The second area concerns day provision. A survey of our day facilities (seven in all) revealed that some were not functioning well and were inappropriately located. Discussions are now taking place about possible resiting. The third need is for separate provision for people suffering from brain damage. Analysis of our statistics revealed that what we were providing for such people was often inappropriate. A proposal for a separate neuro-psychological rehabilitation unit has now been put forward.

DIFFICULTIES

Most of our difficulties stem, paradoxically, from our good practices. By concentrating on good working relationships across the system, with other agencies and with the local community we have tended to spread ourselves a little too thinly. We now need to consolidate our work within the individual units. Direct, informal contact between staff of the units, although efficient, has sometimes resulted in other staff not acquiring the information they should have. We now try to mention all contacts at the weekly meetings. In expanding our service into the community, we have neglected to ensure that there are always enough staff on our own premises. Also, now that many of our former clients have moved on to be resettled in the community, we do not have the capacity to guarantee adequate follow-up. Now that the joint system has been operating for over three years we are finding the range of problems with which Middlewood House caters is widening. Problem drinkers, for instance, necessitate our expanding our specialist skills and liaising with different agencies. It is also not easy to provide continuity of care and good practices when there are staff changes. This has affected us considerably, especially since senior staff, including the consultant psychiatrist and the officer-in-charge at Middlewood House, have left the system.

THE FUTURE

Some of the future developments, such as the new voluntary rehabilitation hostel, Charles Davis House, sponsored by Birmingham Association for Mental Health and run by Colin Grierson, already offer interesting opportunities for co-operation. A similar venture, Flint Green House, to be run jointly by Birmingham Social Services Department and Copec Housing Trust, will open early in 1984. This will cater for the northern, central and eastern

parts of Birmingham, co-ordinating with Highcroft
Hospital on the same principles as Middlewood House
and Hollymoor Hospital.

The Family Unit, currently based at Middlewood
House will become independent in April 1984. It now
has six places for adults and twelve for children,
and is a welcome development from a small project
set up about two years ago for families needing help
with looking after children.

The expansion of the day centre at Middlewood
will continue, with evening social sessions held in
people's own flats. A 'drop-in' service on Sundays
is also planned, and finally, an offshoot centre in
the south of the borough will give social support to
the people in that community instead of their having
to travel to Middlewood

Along different lines, we hope that our new
assessment forms, in conjunction with the
introduction of the nursing process will give a
better service to clients in all units. Finally, in
addition to our invaluable Medidos system, a new
microprocessor-based system will be available for
reminding and recording medication. This, we hope,
will go some way towards reducing readmission rates
for those who forget to take their medication.

Although we are a Joint Demonstration District
we have no access to special additional resources,
so in showing that our approach can work and
continue to develop, we are demonstrating a system
which could be adopted in almost any district in the
country.

REFERENCES

DHSS (1975). Better Services for the Mentally Ill.
    Cmnd 6233, HMSO, London.
DHSS (1983). Health Service Development. Care in the
    Community and Joint Finance.
    Circular HC(83)6/LAC(83)5.

Chapter Sixteen

A WORM'S EYE VIEW: EXPERIENCES AS AN ADMINISTRATOR

Frank Osborn

An administrator with responsibility for non-acute
and community services - the Cinderellas of the NHS
- has particular problems, especially in relation to
securing adequate funding. He also has a privileged
view of things. This worm's eye view derives from
the activities of underpinning, guiding - or, when
necessary, obstructing - a wide variety of proposed
changes to the services, whilst also bearing the
brunt of disappointment when plans fail to mature.
My own view is also unusual in that I was pitched
into the non-acute field - from a background of
local authority health administration - as a result
of problems in the district, and was told simply to
get on with it and sort things out. This gave me a
free hand, but not a lot of guidance. I have, in
consequence, tended to be able to use a fresh
approach to many difficulties and problems.
    From my experience over the last eight years or
so, as District General Administrator in the City
and Hackney Health District, I have put together a
list of items which have influenced my work, and
this chapter discusses some of them, based largely
on the questions put to me during the conference
sessions. The list includes issues involving
national and local policies, the planning and
management structure within which administrators
have to work and the ways in which people
collaborate with me and with each other. It is not a
tidy list, but neither is my job:

- hospital versus community: budgets and
  services;
- sources of money;
- volunteers and voluntary groups;
- jealousies: intra-professional; professional
  and voluntary;

- budgets: functional versus non-functional;
- planning: services, teams, joint planning;
- planning strategies;
- national policies, especially 'Care in the Community';
- the time it takes from planning to implementation;
- career aspirations versus the needs of the service;
- Members' aspirations and pre-conceptions.

Some of these issues have been covered in other chapters; some I propose to discuss further here; others are listed but mentioned only cursorily.

AN ADMINISTRATOR'S ROLE

My main role as an administrator is to talk to and get to know as many people as possible who are concerned with the groups of services for which I am responsible so that I can learn from them how best to help them get what they see as improvements to their services. I regard myself as acting as a bridge in order to break down some of the barriers in the problem areas mentioned above. I also regard it as important for an administrator to be able to suggest innovations, so I have to understand the principles involved in their work. The immediate problem, as recognised by Dr Dick (see Chapter 14), is one of language. Just as the other professions, administrators have their own esoteric language and attitudes which may be far from helpful. Even now, there are some who refer to the mentally ill as 'loonies' and who still feel that they do not deserve humane health care but should be shut away in institutions out in the countryside. I am reconciled to having to accept this attitude from some of my colleagues, but personally believe that any administrator who wants to become better at his job should actually work for a time in all the various groups of services, in order to learn their features, priorities and language. The current (1982) re-organisation of the NHS has been undertaken and vastly manipulated by people who mostly have only ever worked in the acute fields and have, therefore, very little practical knowledge of, or interest in, the non-acute services. Thus lip-service is paid to the value of services like psychiatry, and often that is all it is.
One of the major implications of all the issues which arise in my work is the need for education and

more careful communication. For instance, I refer to
mental illness services as 'non-acute' when clearly
many people have acute mental illnesses. Similarly,
general medicine is labelled 'acute' although many
physical conditions are chronic. This terminology
represents the administrators' shorthand for
distinguishing parts of the budget, but carries no
implications for the type of care. However, it does
cause concern amongst other professions. In my
opinion, it may well be worth attempting to shed the
'non-acute' label for those elements of the
psychiatric service which provide acute care, even
though this will mean being in competition with the
powerful specialties of surgery and general
medicine. From an administrative point of view, to
do this would remove some of the 'second class'
status which detracts from our ability to make
improvements to the care we give. Also it could well
enhance the status of psychiatric patients.

FUNDING

As we know, the health service spends a lot of
money. Locally, about 70 per cent goes on staff
salaries; only something like 4.5 per cent is spent
on non-acute psychiatric services. Nationally, six
per cent goes for capital works, 83 per cent for
revenue expenditure. The problems faced by an
administrator in the tussle between acute and non-
acute services relate to the way mainline funds –
the major form of funding for all services – are
allocated. Each district receives an allocation from
the Exchequer via the regional health authority;
what it then does with it depends on district
priorities. Despite the various re-organisations
within the NHS, districts still tend to follow the
traditional pattern that 'what you have you get
again next year, what you don't have you don't get
unless you can pinch it from somebody else'. It
takes a lot of heaving and pushing to shift
resources (but see Chapter 10 for some hints).
    Like mainline funds, joint finance money comes
from the Exchequer, but by a different route. This
money is made available to the health service in
order to fund projects which are of equal value to
both social and health services; the money is
dispensed jointly by the health and the local
authorities. The DHSS has been developing the joint
finance system over the last few years in an attempt
to work out a satisfactory method of funding the
enormous, and increasing, range of activities which

encompass health, social services and all the other
fields which form part of a comprehensive, community-oriented service. The most recent DHSS arrangements, following an earlier experimental and
consultative period, are described in the circular
**Health Service Development, Care in the Community
and Joint Finance** (DHSS 1983). The main aim is to
provide a structure for transferring money to pay
for schemes which will enable people to move from
long-term hospital care into a community setting.
Funding arrangments vary depending on what is
proposed. By and large the idea is to provide either
funds tapering over a period of 10 to 15 years, or,
in appropriate circumstances, a lump sum or annual
payment from health to local authority in respect of
individuals whose care is transferred from hospital
to community. In addition, there is scope for a
variety of pilot projects covering residential
accommodation, support and day care. As Ken Grant
described in Chapter 10, proposals must be endorsed
by the relevant statutory authorities and channelled
through the Joint Consultative Committee.

One major advantage of the revised timescale,
as opposed to the three to five years of pump
priming allowed originally, is that schemes will
have a much greater degree of security. With the
longer time horizons we will be able to plan
strategically and move away from the shopping list
approach which I mention later. We will also be able
to use most of our energies for running the service
rather than constantly worrying about where next
year's salaries or rent are coming from.

A further advantage is that joint finance money
is safeguarded for services run jointly with local
authorities so that only very rarely can money be
siphoned off for acute services or by marauding
troops from large teaching hospitals.

A further source of large sums of money for
some districts is the Urban Aid programme for areas
coming under the Department of the Environment's
Inner Cities Partnership scheme. I have had many
lengthy sessions with DoE officials, trying to argue
the case for health service projects which they are
happy to fund in principle but which, because of
their different background, they find slightly odd,
even unnecessary. Perhaps their recent study of
special housing needs (Richie J et al. 1983) will
improve the understanding of the relationships
between health, housing and environment and make for
better use of urban aid funds in relation to the
more deprived health fields.

Finally, money can come from trust funds and other research grants, including charitable foundations. In many districts there is money in trust which could be used if desired. The amounts are relatively insignificant, but could nevertheless be helpful to pilot some innovation or top-up funds from another source.

One of the trickier problems is getting money transferred from one budget to another within the NHS. Treasurers have their own ways of looking at the way money is paid out: moving money from one budget head to another involves virement (more shorthand), which is usually difficult, but can be done if there is a good case.

I listed functional versus non-functional budgets as one of the problem areas. In some districts there is an identifiable budget for psychiatry; in others the money for psychiatric services is part of a common pool. I suggest that there is scope for arguing the case for a separate budget. Again, the suggestions made by Ken Grant in Chapter 10 are relevant. There is more education to be done: the members of the District Management Team must be convinced of the needs of psychiatry and confident that the professionals have the ability to make proper plans and carry them through. This applies also to the members of the District Health Authority.

PLANNING

I am quite convinced that no effective development can take place while we rely on the shopping list approach to planning. Yet people continue to put forward long lists of good ideas, regardless of the fact that if the money were provided there is no conceivable way it could be spent in a responsible fashion. There are pros and cons to the idea of planning teams which sift ideas and allocate priorities. In some instances they might well be obstructive, on the other hand they can, as has happened in City and Hackney, give powerful impetus to an agreed plan of development. Much depends on getting that agreement and avoiding the problems of jealousies which featured in my original list. But whatever the planning structure, it pays to have a scheme reasonably well worked out and set out in writing. No committee can be expected to grasp a vague idea and turn it into a workable proposal. It is also a fact of life that if you want something you have to be prepared to 'sell it' and lobby your colleagues, friends and anyone else with influence. In many of our projects we have found it worthwhile to canvas local residents and offer reassurance and information before the official planning machinery takes over.

The question of jealousies and rivalry may be unimportant in some districts but should never be overlooked. A good administrator will try to resolve conflicts and may be in a position to engage in judicious manipulation of timescales and money to ensure equitable results. Often, there is a temptation to push problems away and make excuses because of difficult personalities but one of an administrator's tasks is to perceive likely clashes (the worm's eye view again), and tackle the individual or group either surreptitiously or head-on, depending on circumstances. Make friends and influence people is trite but true.

JOINT PLANNING

Like other contributors, I would like to see separate management teams for services such as psychiatry. Management in this way would greatly enhance the use of the 'Care in the Community' approach and would go some way to achieving the joint planning system which we acknowledge to be the most likely way of developing community-based services spanning health, housing, education and social services.

Joint planning is a concept easier to put on to paper than into practice. I do not feel that joint planning is being used to its full potential; this is partly because we do not employ anyone with a 'joint planning' responsibility, so that often it gets pushed to one side. The joint finance exercise is frequently seen as an acceptable alternative, but my idea of joint planning is much wider than that. It would incorporate the allocation of mainline funds (with functional budgeting) and would seek to develop a fully comprehensive service rather than tinkering around with its separate elements.

One of the problems which confronted me when I began working as a hospital administrator was the long-running battle between hospitals and the community. It is a divisive conflict, particularly when it involves planning teams, where there is an immediately apparent dichotomy between the people with a hospital background and those from local authorities, sometimes with an uneasy Community Health Council or voluntary group member sitting

alongside. With luck, there may be a community
administrator on the team who can bridge the gap; in
my own case experience in a community setting has
been invaluable in understanding different points of
view. In this situation, an administrator must
understand exactly how the system works and must
then educate others to use it properly.

VOLUNTEERS

A whole chapter could be devoted to the question
surrounding volunteers and voluntary groups. The
health service is often frightened of voluntary
bodies because of their relative freedom to experiment and to avoid the stifling bureaucracy of large
organisations. Once again, I feel that this conflict
comes back to language, communication and education.
The health service can learn from voluntary agencies
and in turn they have much to teach.

ADMINISTRATORS

Finally, a word about administrators themselves.
Hospital administration is very hierarchical and
beset by the problems of acute versus non-acute
services. An administrator opting to work in the
non-acute side risks being treated as a second-class
citizen by his colleagues. Some people move into
non-acute services because they care and get
satisfaction from that area; others hope to achieve
promotion but fail to appreciate that it might well
be a dead end as far as their colleagues are
concerned. People may be shunted sideways into non-
acute administration after failing in the acute
services. The same comments are true of community
administration and I would appeal to those with
influence to try and demand something from your
administrators; to realise yourselves, and convey to
others, that working in the field of non-acute
services is a fulfilling career, and just as
demanding of skill and energy as work for acute
services.

REFERENCES

DHSS (1983). Health Service Development. Care in the
    Community and Joint Finance.
    Circular HC(83)6/LAC(83)5.
Richie J, Keegan J & Bosanquet N (1983). Housing for
    mentally ill and mentally handicapped people.
    Department of the Environment, HMSO, London.

Chapter Seventeen

BRINDLE HOUSE - A COMMUNITY MENTAL HEALTH SERVICE IN
PRACTICE

Roger Hargreaves

Brindle House opened its doors in October 1977. The
purpose of this chapter is, firstly, to look at the
principles behind the service and how they were
expressed in the service design; secondly to
highlight the most significant features of the
service; and finally to draw some tentative
conclusions after five years of operation and to
look ahead.
     Brindle House offers a community-oriented
mental health service to a sector of 75,000
population, (one of three in the district), the
boundaries of which extend from the suburbs of
Manchester to the summits of the Peak District. The
age range of the clientele is 16-65, there being
separate services for children and for the over-65s.
The service is based at Brindle House itself, which
is a large Victorian house in the centre of Hyde,
the major town. In addition there is an 14-bed ward
at Tameside General Hospital, four miles outside the
catchment area, which provides inpatient care when
that is required. Limited use is made of 'overflow'
facilities in other hospitals and there is a
'satellite' day centre in Glossop. The staff
complement is roughly 36. Sixteen of our staff work
mainly at Brindle House, which provides most of the
day care, all outpatient facilities and is the main
focus for referrals.
     Brindle House has replaced a conventional
service which was based entirely at Tameside General
Hospital; the other two sectors of Tameside and
Glossop District Health Authority still operate on
the conventional model. It was thus unusual in being
a replacement for a service which already conformed
to a model set out in the 1975 White Paper **Better
Services for the Mentally Ill** , and where distance
from the base hospital had not been a major problem.

The intention was not just to relocate the service physically, but to redesign it as a complete entity starting from a set of principles from which each element of the design would be derived; we were fortunate that local circumstances allowed us to start with virtually a 'blank sheet of paper'. The guiding principles were:

1. That we should work on the assumption that most people referred to us would have 'problems in living' rather than formal illnesses and that the predominant treatment approach should therefore be psychosocial rather than medical.
2. That the service should be as flexible, accessible and informal as possible.
3. That there should be a strong emphasis on day care as an alternative to inpatient care.

From these initial principles a set of operational policies was devised:

1. Self-referral would be possible.
2. Initial assessment and the management of treatment would be shared between the major professions (psychiatry, psychology, social work) on the basis of the most effective division of labour, with no presumption that the psychiatrist had overall authority.
3. The 'major' professions did not have a monopoly of wisdom or of counselling skills and the other staff should be allowed and encouraged to contribute to the limit of their interest and abilities.
4. The staffing mix would be weighted towards the non-medical disciplines.
5. The day care would be part of the 'front-line' of the service and managed by the centre team as a whole.
6. The centre's internal appearance and regime would be as informal and non-medical as possible; those attending the centre would be expected to retain a large measure of responsibility for their own lives.
7. Treatment would be offered, as far as practicable, on the basis of explicit contracts and agreements about the problems to be worked upon, and clients would have access to their own notes.
8. The day-care regime would be 'problem centred' and geared towards active short-term therapy rather than long-term occupation.

9. Drug therapies and inpatient treatment would
   continue to be used, but only when alternatives
   had been considered and excluded.

The centre was a joint project of the then Area
Health Authority and Tameside Social Services
Department, with the initial contribution of the
latter being obtained from joint finance. The
building is jointly owned and running costs are
split on a 50/50 basis, with each authority paying
for its own staff (who also divide up approximately
50/50). The management structure is complex and
divided into four elements.

1. The centre as a whole is managed by a joint
   group of officers of the two authorities, which
   meets quarterly.
2. The building is administered by the Social
   Services Department.
3. The centre is run on a day-to-day basis by the
   entire staff team acting collectively, with no
   internal hierarchy.
4. There are, however, hierarchies within each
   professional group and they are, in turn,
   accountable to line managers outside.

Brindle House could not be described as a
comprehensive service: there are no long-stay beds,
no rehabilitative hostels or workshops, no residential facilities. We do not offer a crisis intervention service, nor do we see our primary function
as being to reduce hospital admissions, though this
has proved to be a useful by-product. I think our
service could best be described as a devolved
community version of a general hospital style
service - referrals come from the same variety of
sources, and much of our time is taken up with
routine practice. There are around 630 referrals per
year; 56 per cent of these are from GPs but a
further 16 per cent are self-referrals. Again,
although it is not the main point of the service, we
do have an 'open door' policy, so that people can
just walk in from the street.
At Brindle House there are three groups of
staff. One group (4.5 social workers, 3.5
psychiatrists, one community psychiatric nurse and
one psychologist) acts as 'key therapists', manning
the duty rota and taking initial referrals. The
second group (4.5 general therapists) runs the day
centre activities, and includes a family support
therapist who works mainly outside the centre with

families with young children. The centre also has
three administrative staff and a cleaner. This level
of staffing is exactly the same as in the other two
sectors of the district which operate conventional
services; it differs only in the mix of skills. The
key therapists divide their time between the centre
and the hospital. Nursing and occupational therapy
staff, to whom we have access, also use the hospital
as their base.

The duty officer sees all walk-in referrals and
also co-ordinates response to emergencies. Other
referrals are allocated at staff meetings. There is
no requirement that any referral be screened by a
doctor and in practice around 50 per cent of
referrals go directly to a social worker, community
nurse or psychologist. Because of this system we
have eight people who can take initial referrals and
this greatly speeds up the process of assessing and
treating our clients. Many of the referrals which
are handled by a non-medical member of the key
therapy team may not be seen by a doctor at any
stage in their 'career' in the service.

In most instances we contact clients initially
by visiting them at home where we try to see all the
family whenever possible. Almost 60 per cent of
people referred are seen the same day, and virtually
all will be seen within 10-15 working days of
referral. If a client needs to be admitted to the
day centre, that can be arranged more or less
immediately since there is no waiting list. At any
one time the team will have around 450 'open' cases,
of whom perhaps 65 will be attending the centre and
12-14 will be inpatients.

Over the years we have come to appreciate some
of the limitations of working as we do. The main
ones seem to be:

1. That the size of the staff team is probably at
   the optimum for operating 'communal management'.
2. That there is a vast latent demand for the sort
   of psychosocial counselling offered by the
   centre and that, as it becomes better known and
   as GP referral habits change, the referral
   rate, currently fairly static, is likely to
   rise again (GP referral rates vary by a factor
   of more than 4 to 1).
3. That the team is 'centre-based' and does not
   have much staff time available for intensive
   work in clients' homes. This limits the extent
   to which inpatient admissions can be prevented.

4. That the centre provides a better service to highly motivated neurotic clients than to those with chronic disabilities, who need facilities such as hostels, sheltered workshops, and unstructured day care which are not available. Attempts have been made to cater for this group within the overall centre programme but these have been frustrated by the problems of the incompatibility of different regimes. Due to the absence of suitable facilities for the more chronic clients there has been a tendency, over the last year or so, for the inpatient beds to begin to 'silt up'.

The team is currently looking at or is working on a number of possible developments, all of which involve the devolution of services away from the centre and closer to the community. Some of these developments have already been piloted. For instance, we are considering running outposted groups in local community centres, or in day nurseries, though this would be at the expense of centre-based activities. We could provide a consultation service to GPs who wish to retain overall responsibility for treatment, with the possibility of sending some of our staff to do sessions in general practice. We would also see great value in setting up an informal 'drop-in' day centre for chronically disabled people, and in increasing the community psychiatric nursing establishment, linking it more closely to Brindle House. Some of us are also closely involved with voluntary groups who are setting up hostel and a sheltered workshop. These would be the first such facilities available in the area.

There have been a number of other persistent problems which have not greatly affected the viability of the service but which should perhaps serve as a warning to others contemplating similar schemes. In particular:

1. It has proved difficult to co-ordinate the regime at Brindle House with that of the ward, which is part of a larger inpatient unit with a different philosophy and different priorities.
2. The two authorities have tended to be reluctant to allow the consultants to relinquish overall responsibility, or to allow 'non- professional' staff to undertake more than limited, practical tasks or to work outside the centre. To some extent there has been a tension between the

social   services tradition in which unqualified
staff often have considerable autonomy, and the
health service tradition in which paramedical
staff work within very restricted boundaries.
3. Both authorities have had some difficulty in
coming to terms with the notion of 'communal
management' and make no secret of their
preference for a hierarchical system with an
'officer-in-charge'.
4. The nursing establishment, in particular, has
been slow to adapt to the different
professional and organisational demands made by
the new service and there is, in consequence, a
danger that nurses will find themselves
relegated to a peripheral role.
5. The long timescale of health service planning
means that hospital-based developments, planned
before the inception of Brindle House, cannot
easily be revised in the light of experience
gained, and work is due to start on a new
'standard mental illness unit' whose facilities
are largely superfluous to the needs of the
Brindle House sector.

During the six years or so since Brindle House
opened the number of 'emergencies' (as measured by
requests from GPs from domiciliary visits) has
fallen by 70 per cent, whilst total referrals have
increased by about 30 per cent. In-patient
admissions have fallen by 40 per cent, and bed
occupancy rate by about 36 per cent, levelling off
in the last three years to rates well below the
national averages. The number of compulsory
admissions is closer to the national average,
reflecting the 'hard core' of people who suffer
acute psychotic breakdowns.
The day centre has a nominal capacity of 35 per
day and at the end of six years it continues to
operate according to its original operational
policy. Such changes as have occurred have been
evolutionary in nature. The collective management
system has functioned well and the transfer of
responsibilities from medical to non-medical staff
has been generally accepted by referring agencies.
The rate of new referrals has levelled off in the
last two years, and it seems probable that the team
is now 'in touch' with the majority of people in the
sector who are vulnerable to repeated breakdowns.
This is our impression from studying the steady
increase in the proportion of self-referrals who are
former clients returning for further help. On the

whole there can be no doubt that Brindle House has
improved the service offered to people with
psychiatric problems and the staff would attribute
the centre's success to four main factors. Firstly,
ease of access for clients, and the rapid response
offered to initial referrals. Secondly, the team's
ability to concentrate a great deal of therapeutic
manpower on a problem in its early stages, and to
marshall its range of skills and abilities to best
advantage. Thirdly, there is a high degree of
congruence between the objectives of client and
therapist and of active participation by the client
in the treatment process. Lastly, there is the ready
availability of day care as an alternative to
inpatient treatment.

The team does not see Brindle House as the
ultimate expression of a community model. In fact,
they think that the centre is fairly close to the
limits of its potential in its present form and that
substantial further progress can be achieved only by
adopting a different model. Some further progress
could, however, be achieved within the present model
if the centre was supported by a network of
satellite facilities.

Chapter Eighteen

PSYCHIATRIC ILLNESS IN GENERAL PRACTICE

Anthony W Clare

INTRODUCTION

In the conditions of the British National Health
Service from its inception, the general practitioner
is the physician of first contact, the professional
figure who is the gatekeeper to all medical
facilities. From the very outset, the service has
been organised around the GP who occupies a central
position in the health service structure, a
structure which differs radically from that
encountered in most other developed countries. Given
that the GP keeps records of his consultations, it
seemed reasonable to researchers in the late 1950s
and early 1960s to try to assess the amount and
nature of the mental disorders with which the GP is
concerned. Initially, however, the prevalence rates
of psychiatric disorders in this setting showed
enormous variation, with referral rates ranging from
17.5 to 160.6 per 10,000 at risk. However, what
seemed to be less variable was the proportion of
patients regarded by the GP as suffering from
psychological problems and referred to a
psychiatrist (Kaeser & Cooper 1971). The finding
that only about 5 per cent of psychiatric patients
presenting in general practice are referred onwards
is one which persists in relevant studies to this
day (Williams & Clare 1981).
   Whereas the psychiatrist and specialist
psychiatric services are primarily concerned with
psychotic illnesses, severe and moderately severe
neurotic disorders and personality disabilities, the
GP is much more concerned with conditions which, if
a diagnostic formulation can be made, fall within
the category of mixed affective disorder, and when a
diagnostic formulation cannot be made with any
confidence, can simply be symptomatically described

as 'anxiety' and/or 'depression' (Clare 1982).

The first systematic study of psychiatric ill-health in general practice was undertaken by Shepherd and colleagues, and involved 46 GPs in London (Shepherd 1966). For each psychiatric case identified in this study, the GPs were asked to record the social factors which they regarded as relevant, in the sense of being implicated in either the onset, course or severity of the patient's illness. Although no factors were specified for a minority of cases, it appeared that in general the doctors regarded social factors as important in the aetiology of psychiatric illness. They tended to report concurrent factors such as marital disharmony, housing problems and work difficulties rather than remote difficulties such as childhood experiences, and there was a surprising conformity of opinion amongst the survey doctors as to which factors were more common and more important. Apart from 'occupational and employment problems', all the social factors were more commonly recorded for female patients and the distribution of the factors varied considerably with age.

PRIMARY CARE MANAGEMENT OF PSYCHIATRIC ILL-HEALTH

Faced with a patient suffering from emotional disorder, the GP has a number of treatment options from which to choose. He can decide to treat the patient himself. He can participate in treatment as part of a multidisciplinary team which may include social workers, psychologists, health visitors, nurses and psychiatrists. He may refer the patient to a psychiatrist.

1. GP Treatment
A combination of drug therapy and reassurance is perhaps the commonest form of general practitioner psychiatric treatment (Shepherd et al. 1966) and it has led to the belief that 'in view of the highest prevalence of psychological distress it is doubtful whether we shall see a fundamental change in medical management' (Lancet 1978). There has been a steady increase in the prescribing of psychotropic drugs over the past 20 years. In England and Wales there was an increase of 19 per cent in the prescribing of these drugs between 1965 and 1970 (Parish 1971), and of eight per cent between 1970 and 1975 (Williams 1981). Whereas there has been a steady rise in the number of antidepressants, tranquillisers and sedatives prescribed, there has been an equally

dramatic fall in the prescribing of amphetamines,
barbiturate hypnotics and appetite suppressants.
There is now much evidence to show that over ten per
cent of the population consumes a psychotropic drug
during any one year and that about 15 per cent of
all prescriptions written by GPs are for psychotropic substances (Williams et al. 1982). All
studies of the characteristics of psychotropic drug
consumers have shown that the prevalence of
consumption is higher among women than among men and
that it increases with age.
     Much psychotropic drug use is short-term
(albeit repetitive) but a proportion of patients are
found to be still receiving drugs many months or
even years after inception. Long-term use gives rise
to much concern, raising issues of dependence and
other adverse effects (Marks 1978, Lader 1981).
Prolonged usage of such drugs has been found to be
associated with increased age, previous psychotropic
drug use, higher levels of psychological morbidity
at the beginning of treatment and, in the case of
women, social problems as perceived by women
(Williams et al. 1982).
     In the primary care setting, there is a paucity
of evidence concerning the efficacy of psycho-
tropics. The absence of operational criteria and
standardisation in relation to such symptoms and
symptom complexes as 'anxiety' and 'depression'
contribute to the difficulties of identifying and
treating them. The argument over the classification
of depression, for example, is hardly an academic
one. It is worth noting that GPs are readily and
regularly criticised for their apparent misuse of
the two classes of psychotropic drugs defined as
antidepressants and anxiolytics. A number of
observers have drawn attention to the tendency of
GPs to use subtherapeutic doses (by the standards of
hospital-based psychiatry at any rate) of
antidepressants (Johnson 1974, Tyrer 1978), to use
antidepressants and anxiolytics interchangeably and
arbitrarily (Weissman & Klerman 1977, Weissman 1981)
and to achieve dispiritingly low levels of drug
compliance on the part of their patients (Rashid
1982).
     The percentage of patients who receive some
form of psychotherapy ranges from 25 per cent in
London practices (Shepherd et al. 1966) to 96 per
cent in industrial dispensaries in Monroe County,
New York (Rosen et al. 1970). However, part of this
variation is almost certainly due to differing ideas
as to what constitutes psychotherapy. Most articles

dealing with psychotherapy in general practice clearly have in mind relatively simple techniques whereby the doctor provides sympathy, advice and/or reassurance (WHO 1973), exercises tolerance and understanding (Kiely 1971, Frank and Frank 1973) and is a good listener (Luban-Plozza 1973).

During recent years, however, there has been considerable interest in the possible adaptation of psychoanalytically-based psychotherapy to meet the needs and realities of general practice. Perhaps the strongest single influence in Western Europe in this regard has been that associated with the name of Michael Balint, and subsequently developed by a number of his colleagues (Balint 1957, Bacla 1971, Balint and Norrell 1976). Balint observed that the most frequently used 'drug' in general practice was the doctor himself, and he believed that the doctor should know how to make optimum use of that drug, to enable him to 'tune into the patients wavelength' within the confines of a short interview. Goldberg, for his part, has drawn attention to the importance of the GP in identifying psychiatric morbidity and treating it efficiently by means of a number of consultation skills andd techniques (Goldberg & Huxley 1980) while there is a growing literature devoted to the potential gains to be anticipated if general practitioners acquire basic counselling skills and a more systematic approach to the provision of advice, reassurance, a sympathetic ear and problem clarification (Ornstein 1977, Sherer & Johnson 1980, Wyld 1981).

2. The Team

Treatment involving the use of drugs and/or psychotherapy may be conducted by the general practitioner acting on his own. The concept of teamwork in general practice covers psychiatrists, community physicians, psychiatrically trained nurses, social workers, psychologists, health visitors as well as GPs themselves. The team, by virtue of its composition, should ideally reflect the multi-faceted nature of the psychosocial problems manifested by patients in the primary care sector. Yet despite the impressive literature testifying to the intermeshed nature of much psychiatric ill-health and social difficulties, the response in terms of the organisation of the appropriate services is far from a co-ordinated one. While general practitioners are independent con-tractors to the National Health Service, the social services are administered by the local authorities.

The Seebohm Report, which was crucially influential regarding the decision that each local authority should establish a social service department, did emphasise the need for liaison between the general medical and social services. 'We regard teamwork between general practitioners and social workers as vital', the Report declared. 'It is one of our main objectives and the likelihood of promoting it is a test we would like to see applied to our proposals for a social service department.'

In terms of such a test, however, it is hard to contest the view that the Seebohm proposals have not been entirely successful. At the time of the Report, there was considerable evidence of the lack of liaison between general practitioners and social workers (Harwin et al. 1970), a state of affairs later confirmed by a national survey of Area Directors of Social Services (Ratoff et al. 1973) which revealed that while the Seebohm Committee had recommended that social workers be specifically attached to GPs, only 1.5 per cent of social workers in the country were actually deployed in this fashion.

Since then, however, the situation has somewhat improved and the literature is replete with reports of various kinds of attachment liaison schemes involving the two professional groups (Cooper 1971, Gilchrist et al. 1978, Corney 1980). Yet the relationship is far from that envisaged by Seebohm to judge by the comments of social workers responding to researchers investigating the social work task (Parsloe & Stevenson 1978). The general practitioner was seen as someone with little knowledge of what social workers did, who was critical of the professional standing of social work and treated social workers in a patronising fashion. While caution must be exercised in interpreting what is little more than anecdote and opinion, it is interesting to note that those social workers who were more favourably inclined towards GPs were working within some form of attachment arrangement in the primary care setting.

Social workers, in common with other professionals in the health service, appear unaware of the remarkable organisational and educational developments which have been underway in general practice during the past 15 years. Such changes will, it must be conceded, take time to work through to affect the standard and quality of primary care in general but they are, nonetheless, changes which have potential implications for the involvement of

social workers, and other health care professionals
in primary care. The growth of the multidisciplinary
health centre is one such development. In the five
years between 1972 and 1977, the number of health
centres in England and Wales rose from 212 to 713
and the Royal Commission on the Health Service
estimated that there would be 900 by the end of the
1970s and 1000 by the early 1980s. At the present
time, if one includes multi-partner group practices
in premises owned and run by GPs themselves, it can
be estimated that at least one in four GPs works in
a health centre defined in a recent DHSS circular as
'premises provided by an area health authority where
primary health care services are provided by general
practitioners, health visitors and district nurses
and possibly other professions'.

The reference to 'other professions' may appear
somewhat tentative. It may also be a recognition of
the ambivalent position adopted by the social work
profession towards primary care in general. It is of
course true that social work faces heavy demands
particularly in the areas of child care and the
provision of social services to the elderly and the
handicapped. But it is doubtful that the enormity of
the current social work load is the only or the
complete explanation for the persistence of the
split in the provision of psychosocial care between
the primary care and social services. It is also
true that many GPs, particularly older ones and
those accustomed to working single-handedly, are not
particularly enamoured by the notion of working in a
collective team exercise with social workers, or
indeed with other professionals. There is widespread
criticism too, within the medical profession, of the
allegedly low level of knowledge and expertise
relating to physical and mental ill-health possessed
by post-Seebohm social workers (BMJ 1980, Brewer &
Lait 1980) which undoubtedly militates against
closer collaboration.

It may well be that these various obstacles
will serve to frustrate the growth of social worker-
GP collaboration from the experimental and largely
ad hoc attachment schemes scattered throughout the
country to a comprehensive primary care social
service and health collaborative programme. There
are signs that many GPs are able and willing to turn
to other professionals within the primary care team,
most notably the health visitor and the district
nurse, for assistance in the management of
psychosocial disorders. Whether this is an
appropriate solution is a question which social

workers might be expected to address themselves to
and answer over the coming decade. But it is
difficult to ignore the fact that the opportunity
for social work as a profession to play a more
significant role in the develoment of the primary
care service has never been more obvious than at the
present time. In addition to the operational
developments which make it physically easier to
locate other professionals alongside the GP, there
are developments in the vocational training of
general practitioners (Pereira Gray 1979, RCGP
1979), a growing realisation concerning the need for
a more appropriate range of therapeutic responses to
the demands of psychosocial disorders (Clare & Lader
1982) and a greater awareness of the shortcomings in
the quality and competence of the primary care
services at the present time (Cartwright & Anderson
1981) which, taken together, all underline the need
and the opportunity for professionals with social
knowledge and skills to be deployed within primary
care.

3. The Role of the Psychiatrist

According to a recent review (Williams 1979), young
patients, males and psychotics are more likely to be
referred to psychiatrists by GPs. Brook (1978) put
forward what he considered to be the four main
reasons for referral:

1. The general practitioner wants an expert
   opinion so that he can himself continue
   treatment armed with this expert knowledge.
2. The general practitioner wants the
   psychiatrists to provide or arrange specialist
   treatment that he cannot provide himself.
3. The general practitioner wants to share the
   burden of and responsibility for one of his
   patients for whom little can be done.
4. The general practitioner wants to be relieved
   of the patient for a while.

Brook points out that the first two reasons are
primarily in the interests of the patient, and that
the last two are primarily in the interests of the
doctor. Kaeser and Cooper (1971) investigated a
sample of patients referred to the outpatients
department and the emergency clinic at the Maudsley
Hospital. As well as obtaining information from the
records, they interviewed as far as possible the
referring doctors and the referred patients.
    The GPs rarely considered the need for diag-

nosis and a specialised opinion to be the main reason for referral, and in the majority of cases they
wanted the hospital to take over responsibility.
Requests for special investigation and treatment
were also rare, and indeed such investigations were
rarely performed. No patient in the sample was sent
to the clinical psychology department, and only one
to the EEG department. The findings of Johnson
(1973), in his study of outpatient services at
Manchester, were somewhat different. He found that a
diagnostic opinion was required in 63 per cent of
referrals, and that special investigations were
thought necessary by the referring practitioner for
46 per cent of the patients. In direct contrast to
the findings of Kaeser and Cooper, the Manchester
GPs in about 50 per cent of cases wanted 'advice
only - with treatment to be continued by the family
doctor'.

These disparate findings point to a wide range
of opinion among GPs about what they want from the
psychiatrist, and unfortunately these needs are
rarely made explicit in the referral letter. As
Brook (1978) points out, 'if the psychiatrist does
not perceive the real reason for the referral ...
the general practitioner can feel as let down by the
psychiatrist as the patient feels let down by him.
The general practitioner finishes up with feelings
of frustration towards the clinic and is often less
able to help his patient.'

Three other important reasons for referral
emerged from Kaeser & Cooper's (1971) study. In the
emergency clinic referrals, the presence of
behaviour disturbance, serious social problems or
the possibility of suicidal risk were regarded as
important. For both outpatient and emergency clinic
referrals, 'failure to respond to general practitioners treatment', and 'patient request for specialist referral' were frequently given as the main
reason for referral.

The frequency of patient request is of
particular importance, as it underlines the fact
that in a substantial proportion of cases it is the
patient himself rather than the doctor who
determines referral - a finding confirmed by Johnson
(1973). This is also similar to the results of
Richards (1960), who reviewed a series of referrals
to the Maudsley Hospital and found that about one-
third had been initiated by the patient himself or
by a relative. Likewise, Rawnsley & Loudon (1962) in
their study in South Wales found that pressure from
relatives was an important influence on referral.

One of the most important implications of this research was summarised by Kaeser & Cooper (1971) as follows: '(there is) an absence of firmly established clinical indications .... the selection of cases for specialist care is heavily influenced by non-clinical factors'. This may point to the need for a reorientation of the basic model of clinical psychiatric practice. Although there is an absence of 'firmly established clinical indications' for referral, the evidence points strongly to a close relationship between the extent of the problem posed by the patient and referral. Patients cause problems for the GP - that is, they do not respond to treatment - and hence they are referred; patients cause problems to relatives and perhaps to the community in general, and hence are referred; patients regard themselves as having a problem, and hence ask for a referral. Williams (1979) reviews evidence to suggest that improvements might result from psychiatrists adopting a problem-oriented, rather than the traditional diagnosis-oriented, approach to patient management.

There is evidence that general practitioners are not greatly enamoured by the service they receive from psychiatrists. In the Kaeser & Cooper study, about 55 per cent of the GPs thought that referral had been helpful and that outcome had broadly matched expectations but in 15 per cent of cases the GPs felt that little or nothing had been achieved by referral. The attitudes of patients were similar. Whereas nearly 60 per cent of the patients thought they had been helped, a substantial minority of patients (26 per cent) felt they had received no benefit while the remainder were unable or unwilling to express an opinion.

One important influence on the general practitioner's perception of a psychiatric service is the adequacy of communication between him and the psychiatrists. At the present time, face-to-face discussions are limited (Williams 1979) and virtually the only channels of communication are the referral letter and the reports back to the GP (Long & Atkins 1974). It has been suggested that a different model of GP-psychiatrist interaction might be more appropriate. Some favour the psychiatrist seeing a greater proportion of psychiatrically distressed patients than the five to ten per cent he sees at the present time. An alternative model envisages the psychiatrist playing a greater role as a teacher and educator who aims to improve the GPs skills in recognising and treating psychiatric

disorder without recourse to specialist referral. A
third approach involves the psychiatrist working out
in the community as a member of the
multidisciplinary primary care team.

SUMMARY

Psychiatrists clearly have a role in educating
general practitioners but there is an equivalent
role for GPs in making psychiatrists better informed
about the 90 per cent of psychiatric morbidity which
they never see. Too often psychiatrists talk of
community psychiatry without paying much attention
to the very system, namely the primary care service,
which the World Health Organisation regards as 'the
cornerstone of community psychiatry' (WHO 1973). The
provision of an integrated, comprehensive and
efficient mental health service depends on the
recognition by the hospital-based services of the
role played by primary care personnel, the burden of
morbidity currently carried by them and the crucial
role relating to referral and utilisation of the
specialist services played by the primary health
care team and, in particular, by the general
practitioner.

REFERENCES

Bacal H (1971). Training in psychological medicine:
an attempt to assess Tavistock Clinic seminars.
Psychiatry in Medicine, 2, pp 13-22.
Balint E & Norrell J S (1976). Six Minutes for the
Patient: Interactions in General Practice
Consultation. Tavistock, London.
Balint M (1957). The Doctor, His Patient and the
Illness. Pitman Medical, London.
Brewer C & Lait J (1980). Can Social Work Survive?
Temple Smith, London.
British Medical Journal (1980). Prescription for
social work. Editorial, 2, pp 890-891.
Brook A (1978). An aspect of community mental
health: consultative work with general practice
teams. Health Trends 10, pp 37-39.
Cartwright A & Anderson R (1981). General Practice
Revisited. Tavistock, London.

Clare A W (1982). Problems of Psychiatric Classification in General Practice, in Psychiatry and General Practice, edited by A W Clare and M Lader. Academic Press, London.

Clare A W & Lader M (1982). Psychiatry and General Practice. Edited proceedings of Mental Health Foundation Conference, Oxford, 1981. Academic Press, London.

Cooper B (1971). Social work in general practice: the Derby scheme. Lancet i, pp 539-542.

Corney R H (1980). Factors affecting the operation and sucess of social work attachment schemes in general practice. Journal of the Royal College of General Practitioners, 30, pp 149-158.

Frank I & Frank R K (1973). Problems of sexuality as encountered in a general family practice. Psychosomatics, 14, pp 230-232.

Gilchrist I C, Gough J B, Horsfall-Turner Y R, Ineson E M, Keele G, Marks B & Scott H J (1978). Social work in general practice. Journal of the Royal College of General Practitioners, 28, pp 675-679.

Goldberg D & Huxley P (1980). Mental Illness in the Community. Tavistock, London.

Harwin B G, Cooper B, Eastwood M R & Goldberg D P (1970). Prospects for social work in general practice. Lancet, ii, pp 559-561.

Johnson D (1973). A further study of psychiatric outpatient services in Manchester. An operational study of general practitioner and patient expectation. British Journal of Psychiatry, 123, pp 185-191.

Johnson D A W (1974). A study of the use of antidepressant medication in general practice. British Journal of Psychiatry, 125, pp 186-192.

Kaeser H C & Cooper B (1971). The psychiatric patient, the general practitioner, and the outpatient clinic: an operational study and a review, Psychological Medicine, vol 1, pp 312-325.

Kiely W F (1971). Psychotherapy for the family physician. American Family Physician, 3, pp 87-91.

Lader M (1981). Benzodiazepine Dependence, in The Misuse of Psychotropic Drugs, edited by R Murray et al. Special Publication No 1, Gaskell Publications, Royal College of Psychiatry.

Lancet (1978). Stress, distress and drug treatment. Editorial, 4, pp 1347-1348.

Long A & Atkins J B (1974). Communications between general practitioners and consultants. British Medical Journal, 4, pp 456-459.

Luban-Plozza B (1973). Preventive medicine and psychological aspects of family practice. Psychiatry in Medicine, 3, pp 327-332.

Marks J (1978). The Benzodiazepines: Use, Overuse, Misuse, Abuse. MTP Press, Lancaster.

Ornstein P (1977). The family physician as a 'therapeutic instrument'. Journal of Family Practice, 4, p 659.

Parish P O (1971). The prescribing of psychotropic drugs in general practice. Journal of the Royal College of General Practitioners, 21, supplement 4, pp 1-77.

Parsloe P & Stevenson O (1978). Social Service Teams: The Practitioner's View, DHSS; HMSO.

Pereira Gray D G (1979). A System of Training for General Practice. Occasional Paper No 4, Royal College of General Practitioners, London.

Rashid A (1982). Do patients cash prescriptions? British Medical Journal, 284, p 24.

Ratoff L, Cooper B & Rockett D (1973). Seebohm and the NHS: a survey of medico-social liaison. British Medical Journal (Suppl), 2, pp 51-53.

Rosen B M, Locke B Z, Goldenberg I D & Babigan H M (1970). Identifying emotional disturbance in persons seen in industrial dispensaries. Mental Hygiene, 54, pp 271-279.

Royal College of General Practitioners (1979). Trends in General Practice. RCGP, London.

Shepherd M, Cooper B, Brown A C & Kalton G (1966). Psychiatric Illness in General Practice. OUP, London.

Sherer L M & Johnson A H (1980). Resident development in family practice training: a personal counselling programme. Journal of Family Practice, 10, pp 1017-1023.

Tyrer P (1978). Drug treatment of psychiatric patients in general practice. British Medical Journal, 2, pp 1008-1010.

Weissman M M (1981). Depression and its treatment in a US urban community, Archives of General Psychiatry, 38, pp 417-421.

Weissman M M & Klerman G L (1977). The chronic depressive in the community - unrecognised and poorly treated. Comprehensive Psychiatry, 18, pp 523-532.

Williams P (1981). Trends in the Prescribing of Psychotropic Drugs, in The Misuse of Psychotropic Drugs, edited by R Murray et al. Special Publication, No 1, Gaskell Publications, Royal College of Psychiatrists.

Williams P (1979). The Interface between Psychiatry and General Practice. SK & F Publications, 2.

Williams P & Clare A (1981). Changing patterns of psychiatric care. British Medical Journal, 282, pp 375-377.

Williams P, Murray J & Clare A (1982). A longitudinal study of psychotropic drug prescription. Psychological Medicine, 12, pp 201-206.

World Health Organisation (1973). Psychiatry and Primary Medical Care. WHO, Copenhagen.

Wyld K L (1981). Counselling in general practice: a review. British Journal of Guidance and Counselling, 9, pp 129-141.

Chapter Nineteen

DAY HOSPITAL FOR DEMENTIA: SAFETY NET FOR A HIGH-
WIRE ACT?

Susan Hodgson

I work with a psychogeriatric service in south
Manchester which serves a district of about 200,000
people. The service includes an excellent social
work team and a team of five community psychiatric
nurses, both with no other commitments. We have
about 25,000 elderly in our health district so we
need to contribute help for some of the 2,500 or so
demented people in our community, of whom we
estimate half will be fairly severely disabled. We
are trying to be available to GPs, families and
social services to help with those people, and that
includes helping people to cope with the client,
wherever he may be. We certainly do not wish to
claim all those people as our own or insist that the
hospital services alone should deal with them. We
are unusual in that we have never inherited any
long-stay geriatric patients from a mental hospital.
The long-stay facilities have grown up with the
service, and we have relatively few long-stay beds.
    We have two wards with about 20 beds in each,
in two different hospitals. We also run long-term
continued-care supported day hospitals for demented
patients in conjunction with each long-stay ward,
which is something I have not seen elsewhere. It
grew out of necessity initially because the only
building available was the the original lunatic
asylum for the workhouse, which was eventually given
to us, refurbished and became the new
psychogeriatric unit. The ground floor is the ward
for long-stay patients and we made an ad hoc day
hospital within the ward. So day patients came and
shared exactly the same ward space as the
inpatients, and the day hospital nursing staff
worked alongside the long-stay nursing staff. We
find that there are great advantages in this system,
because knowledge of the two groups of staff about

patients is shared and co-operation between the two
groups is tremendous. If a day patient is ill and
needs rescuing for a few days, the inpatient nursing
staff already know him and the day nursing staff do
not feel that they have lost a patient to a ward
miles away. Also, the same staff, the same
occupational therapists, physiotherapists and
medical staff are servicing the whole group of
patients, so there is an enormous amount of
information immediately available.

When the day hospital to accompany the other
ward became possible we created the same set-up,
although the day hospital was more generously
provided with facilities, with some of its own
rooms, particularly for nursing operations and
administration. We used the same model, so that the
day patients would come in and share the space and
the activities, meals and so on, with inpatients.
One advantage is that it structures the week for the
inpatients and staff, which is hard to do in long-
stay situations. It also creates a more vital
atmosphere on the ward, in that on weekdays lots of
people arrive in hats and coats, take them off, have
cups of tea, exchange news and join in activities.
Life seems much nearer to normal, and much more
interesting for all concerned. Each of those units
provide about fifteen day places per day. Most
people come more than once a week, probably on
average two days a week.

The day hospital is not intended to be an
assessment centre, a short-term rehabilitation
centre, or a step towards inpatient care, it is
intended to be a continuing care module. Obviously
for some patients it may prove to be a step towards
some other end, but for most its function is to
sustain them and their families for as long as
necessary, and when they die it is likely they will
die at home.

Obviously these are not the only facilities for
the confused elderly. Manchester has a very strong
tradition of good social services provision,
particularly for the mentally ill and the elderly
since the last war, so that residential places for
the elderly are well up to the national norm. There
is a lot of enthusiasm and concern about maintaining
a good domiciliary service available to everybody,
particularly the elderly. So although we have
suffered from the expenditure cuts, the squeezes on
home help provision, meals on wheels etc., we did
start from a relatively privileged position. Area
social workers may not be able now to give as much

time as they would like to some cases, which causes
dissatisfaction and difficulty. One of the dangers
of a reasonable system is complacency, and now, more
than ever, it is extremely important to evaluate new
developments and services.
     One of the developments in our area is that
most of the 14 old people's homes in our health
district take some people for day care, as long as
they do not have major behavioural problems. We
would like to develop day care in residential homes,
and make them mini-resource centres for their local
community. Psychogeriatricians such as ourselves
have strong links with the homes, doing
consultations about patients in the homes, taking
some residents as inpatients, and some of our own
patients are admitted to homes. We try to encourage
this interaction. Homes should be better treated by
the services, particularly the health service. At
the moment, when someone is put in a home it may be
assumed that his or her needs will be met and staff
will be able to cope - they are left to themselves.
The staff are often doing immensely hard work, with
very little support or expertise. We are
continuously being asked for advice by these people,
so it would obviously be extremely helpful if the
hospital services - physiotherapists, occupational
therapists and community psychiatric nurses - could
spend time contributing to the care in the homes.
     It is hardly surprising that the elderly take
up a lot of health service time due to the multiple
nature of their problems. However, the pattern of
provision varies between health districts. In my
district, the social services, the geriatric and
psychogeriatric departments all contribute to care
for the elderly mentally ill. In other districts,
one or other of these services may be underdeveloped
or may not exist. Although it is relatively easy to
find out the type of provisions made by each
district, there is little knowledge available about
the characteristics of the population served. Some
recent research carried out in our district has shed
some light on this (Charlesworth & Wilkin 1982). The
research team collected information about 822 people
cared for in the various facilities. Using a simple
behavioural scale, data were collected from
relatives or members of staff who were familiar with
the patient. Items covered included mobility,
orientation, communication, co-operation, rest-
lessness, dressing, feeding, continence, bathing and
memory function. The findings of the study showed
that three significant patterns emerged which

correlated   with   the   way demented people should be
allocated   between   psychiatry,   social services and
geriatrics. Thus geriatricians were caring for   some
people   with   confusion   and dementia but mainly for
those   with   grave   physical   difficulties.   The
psychogeriatricians   cared   for   those   who   were
globally more disabled. Their   population   was   very
physically   dependent in all respects even though it
was fairly mobile. Of course, the   mental   state   of
these   patients   was worse than in the other groups.
Those people in residential homes·were fairly mobile
and there was a much lower incidence of physical and
mental   problems.   Nevertheless,   there   was   a
significant   incidence   of   people with quite severe
dementia or quite severe physical problems.
     Our social services colleagues may be concerned
because within their own accommodation for   elderly
people   (Part III   accommodation),   they   had   more
people, in total, who had the sort of problems   that
are   normally   seen   in   hospital,   than   were   in
recognised psychogeriatric long-stay beds. This does
not   mean   that   someone is necessarily misplaced by
being in the home; I think there is a lot to be said
for   not   segregating   all   the   seriously   confused
people out of the residential care system. But it is
important   to   recognise   that   the residential care
system therefore needs   a   lot   of   input,   support,
information,   sympathy   and   appreciation   from   the
health services. This study   was   repeated   annually
between   1977   and   1981 in order to see what trends
developed.   There   was   little   change   in   the
characteristics   of   the population in the different
settings. There   was   a   change   with   people   being
slightly   older   on   admission   to   any   of   the
facilities. Hence the admission cohort   was   getting
slightly older and obviously the resident cohort was
getting even older than it is now, and in   addition,
in   the   homes   it   looked   as if people were just a
little bit less able on admission than they   were   a
few years ago. Thus, if people on admission are more
disabled, in a couple of   years'   time   the   characteristics   of   the   longer- term residents will have
altered. This   will   make   the   work   of   the   staff
increasingly difficult unless there are very careful
admission policies and deliberate plans to   maintain
a   tolerable   mixture   of people within the homes. In
order to achieve such a   balance,   collaboration   is
necessary   within   the   social services system itself
and across services.
     Regarding   day   care,   it   is   important   to be
vigilant about the inter-dependency of the different

services. As I mentioned, there are two small
psychogeriatric day hospitals. The geriatric service
has an enormous day hospital, whose emphasis is on
rehabilitating people particularly with mobility and
self-care problems. Its objective is to rehabilitate
them and then discharge them. Thus it is not a
continuing care facility. There are two local
authority day care centres, one exclusively for the
elderly and the other for a mixture of physically
handicapped people, people with psychiatric
problems, and the elderly. There is also day care
provided within the residential homes. It is
difficult to predict future needs. However it seems
to me that there are reasons for trying to monitor
what population we are dealing with in our
psychogeriatric day hospitals, and it is very
important to know which parts of the service are
doing how much work for a particular group of
clients. This needs to be monitored over time
because it is important to know how people are going
to respond on the one hand to the current idealogies
about community care and on the other hand to the
practical problems involved in the transfer of staff
and money and enthusiasm into the community. It is
necessary that we avoid the pitfall of assuming
change has occurred when nothing at all has
happened. The danger is that the voluntary sector
will be relied on to provide services which are
beyond its scope and remit.

From my point of view, the object of day
hospital care for demented people should be to help
those people carry on living independently in the
way that they choose within their part of the
community. In a way it is an extension of
domiciliary support. It is supporting the home in a
wider sense, very often supporting the relatives,
friends and the locality in a meaningful way,
maintaining co-operation and tolerance and providing
a considerable amount of physical care and
behavioural rehabilitation without actually having
to admit someone to hospital. However, it is not the
only way that day care can be used. For instance it
can be used as a holding operation pending long-stay
inpatient care. Here the objective is to keep the
pressure off the hospital and to protect the level
of bed occupancy. Another use may be to solve the
problems of a system that is inadequate both in
terms of inpatient facilities and the domiciliary
support. I would argue that it is important to be
able to establish whether the running of a day
hospital has shifted from a purely patient-oriented

perspective to protecting a bad health care system.

When patients are admitted to our day hospital
we could administer the behavioural screen test that
I mentioned earlier, and which is initially
administered to patients in their homes. This gives
us a behavioural record on first contact with the
patient and a further record when they come in to
the day hospital system. This provides a basis for
comparison. The behavioural screen test can be
repeated annually also, and it is important to
revise information about each 'patient's marital
status, where they live, their accommodation, with
whom they live and perhaps include a comment about
physical abilities or disabilities. It is
particularly important to establish changes in the
patient's living circumstances because a change can
indicate a need for more care even though his mental
state may not be altered. For instance, if a
demented lady's husband suffers a heart attack, it
is probably unreasonable to place as much strain on
him as before. Ideally, we require an annual census
on all the other day care establishments in the
district, so that we can monitor the characteristics
of day patients being cared for by the health
system, the social services system and the private
sector.

To sum up, I have emphasised the need to
establish objectively the way we work and the
characteristics of the population we serve because
as clinicians we are liable, because of the
pressures on our time, to lose sight of such matters
when making decisions about offering day care.

REFERENCE

Charlesworth A & Wilkin D (1982). Dependency among
   old people in geriatric wards, psychogeriatric
   wards and residential homes, 1977-1981. Research
   Report Number 6, University Hospital of South
   Manchester, Psychogeriatric Unit - Research
   Section.

PART FOUR

CONSOLIDATION: LOOKING TO THE FUTURE

Chris Heginbotham's main chapter in the final section covers a good deal of ground. He suggests a list of general principles, examines changes in planning and financing mental health services which would enable local services to be developed, and makes proposals about statutory and non-statutory intervention which could facilitate progress.

It is fitting that Dr Douglas Bennett, chairing one of his last conferences before retirement, should have the final word. His message is one of optimism - that the 'Cinderella' image has finally been vanquished - and relief, that the idea of locally-based services being both possible and preferable has now taken firm root.

Chapter Twenty

THE MYTH OF SISYPHUS: TURNING MOUNTAINS INTO MOLEHILLS

Chris Heginbotham

Sisyphus was condemned by the Gods forever to roll a boulder to the top of a mountain and when he reached the top the boulder would be kicked back to the bottom and he would have to start rolling to the top again. Trying to build a mental health service is rather like the task Sisyphus was set - every time we think we are progressing, the boulder is kicked back to the bottom of the mountain and we have to start all over again. We have all been involved some time or other in trying to build a comprehensive mental health service and we have all met tremendous frustrations in trying to make any change. The voluntary sector, those in the statutory services, and members of health and local authorities work hard to find solutions to push the boulder up the mountain, only to be repulsed by central or local government, by planning regulations or by the system.

THE MAIN CHALLENGES

Principles for a blueprint
We urgently need a comprehensive local mental health service blueprint. That blueprint should set out the broad range of services needed locally with some guidance as to the way that such a service would be implemented. It is not suggested that such a blueprint would be implemented in the same way in each district nor that every element would be required in each locality. We start from a different base in different areas, with different needs, and different hurdles. But it is essential that we have a clear framework for future implementation and that this is based on agreed principles for the type of service we want to see.

We require principles of ordinariness and
'normalisation' appropriate to the needs of sick and
recovering mentally ill people. The principles of
'normalisation' were developed particularly for
mental handicap services, though Wolfensberger in
his original book (1972) also related these
principles to mental health services generally. Dr
Donald Dick, in Chapter 14, describes the way that
such a service might be developed from those
principles, on the idea of 'ordinariness' and the
needs of individuals. We must start to look at
services by considering individuals first and
building up from their needs, rather than starting
with the large hospitals and thinking of ways of
moving parts of them hospitals into the community.
In other words, we need a 'bottom up' approach to
planning rather than the superimposed 'top down'
approach that has traditionally been used. A local
service, then, is one which:

- values the client as a full citizen with rights
  and responsibilities entitled to have an active
  opportunity to influence relevant services, no
  matter how severe the disability;
- aims to promote the greatest self-determination
  of the individual;
- aims to provide and evaluate a programme of
  treatment, care and support based on the needs
  of the individual, regardless of age or
  severity of disability;
- aims to help the client to as ordinary a life
  as possible on the basis of realistic, informed
  choice;
- aims to meet special needs arising from
  disability through a local, accessible, fully
  co-ordinated multidisciplinary service given by
  appropriately trained staff;
- is delivered wherever possible to the client's
  home or usual environment;
- plans actively for people now living in
  institutions to return to the locality and use
  its services if they wish;
- aims to enhance the collective capacity to cope
  with, or alleviate distress.

In addition to the principle of ordinariness we
need to consider the rights of individual patient,
client or consumer. Work is underway in various
areas to consider the 'rights thesis' approach to
the provision of services. Such an approach looks at
the rights of individuals to positive freedoms - the

freedom to choose services and the freedom to refuse
services. Clearly, this takes us into the area of
the legal framework of mental health services. It is
not for a moment suggested that there are not
patients who require treatment but who may be unable
to recognise this fact. It is necessary to recognise
that the step forward in rights for patients, as
partially enshrined in the Mental Health Act 1983,
is important not just because the Act strengthened
the rights of patients, but because this is a
fundamental element in the development of a
comprehensive service for the future. It is sad that
there has been so much antagonism to many of the
proposals within that Act, but hopefully, as the
dust settles, we can begin to develop comprehensive
service on the foundation of the new legal
framework.

Thirdly, we need to consider the position of
mentally ill people in society and to develop a
political economy of mental health. There are
serious inequalities in the types of services
provided for mentally ill people when compared to
services in physical medicine: the Black Report
(1980) on inequalities and health hardly mentions
the subject of mental illness or mental health
services; Lesley Doyal's excellent book (Doyal 1981)
mentions mental health only two or three times, and
much other writing also skirts round the mental
health issue. We need a political economy of mental
health because we must have a clear socio-economic
framework as well as a legal framework for
development of better services. If we are not clear
as to what we are trying to achieve in developing a
comprehensive local mental health service then we
will end up with further confusion as to the type of
service we require. We must come to some agreement
on the aims and objectives of such a service, both
in general terms nationally, and in specific areas
locally.

Taking these three approaches we can develop a
comprehensive local mental health service blueprint
on the basis of individual needs; and this will give
a much better idea of how it will fit in with
existing provision and current ideas for the
development of services.

Education for mental health
Hand in hand with the development of a comprehensive
service blueprint must go a major public mental
health education approach. MIND must work with
statutory and voluntary services locally and with

agencies such as the Health Education Council to develop a major campaign to educate the public in mental health issues. There is still much fear and misunderstanding of mental health and mental illness; if we are to make any headway in the development of a comprehensive service then we have to persuade the general public that mental health services are a high priority and that people should not be overly concerned at the placement of ex-patients in housing or the setting up of hostels, day centres, sheltered workshops and clinics in each locality. A public mental health education programme demands that all of us work together and it demands that we do so fairly urgently. Now is not the time for protracted debate as to whether this has to be done: if we are to make any real progress in the development of a proper service then a concentrated and co-ordinated approach is required.

Preventive measures
The other major challenge goes hand in hand with a public mental health programme and that is prevention. If we are able to run a good public education programme then we are one step nearer preventing some forms of mental illness. Greater awareness of mental health issues and the sorts of reasons for people becoming mentally ill can only be a step in the right direction to a more mentally healthy society. There are however six specific areas that should be of current concern. These are:

- isolation of single parent families;
- the needs of informal carers of elderly mentally infirm people in the community;
- the effects of bad housing on mental health;
- ways of teaching teachers techniques for developing positive mental health education in schools;
- stress at work and ways in which we can take stress out of work, or educate workers, unions and management to minimise stress and its effects;
- unemployment and its effect on psychiatric morbidity.

All of these areas are difficult and demanding and require a lot of hard work. It is to be hoped that various agencies will take up the challenge to consider one or other of these areas and see what preventive measures can be taken and how successful those measures are.

Implementation

It is, of course, all very well to develop a
blueprint for the sort of services we would like to
see. It is another matter to implement such a
blueprint. This is where the mountains suddenly
appear. We need the blueprint but we also need an
agreement to put it into practice. This can be done
if people want to do it; the pessimists who say it
is all too big or too difficult should be rejected.
History is littered with individuals who have 'cried
wolf', who have lacked imagination or drive, or for
whom it was just too difficult. Yet history is
dotted with major achievements. We are capable of
putting men on the moon, or, a bit less exciting and
a bit nearer home, we are capable of building a
major barrage across the Thames. We are capable of
organising, in fourteen days, to fight a war 8,000
miles away from the shores of this island. Indeed,
we can even find the money for this. If we can do
those things then we can also agree together a
programme for comprehensive local mental health
services and we it can be implemented.
     There is no doubt, however, that current NHS
planning systems are complex and fit badly to local
authority systems. The whole is complicated, time-
consuming and wasteful. Recent government re-
organisations have created yet further anomalies,
particularly over boundaries. There are now more
instances on non-coterminosity between health and
local authorities than there were before re-
organisation. If the statistics are right, Bath
District Health Authority takes the prize for being
the one which overlaps with most other authorities,
being non-coterminous with three county authorities
and six district councils. Sadly there is no point
in suggesting further changes at this time. On
current form there will be another re-organisation
in 1990 anyway! What is needed now, and for the next
five years, is a planning framework to develop local
services within the organisation or boundaries that
exist. A framework is needed which will facilitate
the rundown of large psychiatric hospitals and good
collaboration between the NHS, local authorities and
the voluntary sector.

STEPS IN THE PROCESS

I would now like to set out what I see as the ideal
requirements in the implementation of a
comprehensive service. However, it is important to
recognise that not all of these will be possible

immediately in all districts, though there should be
progress towards them wherever possible.

Management
The first step is that every district health
authority should aim to have a psychiatric services
management unit. It may well be too late in many
districts to develop such a structure, since the
current NHS bureaucracy is very much dominated by
individual hospitals, and it seems very difficult
for individual districts to consider putting all
psychiatric services (or, for that matter, maternity
services or those for elderly people) together in
one management unit. The Nodder Committee report in
1978 proposed having psychiatric services management
teams which would cover the long-stay hospital,
general hospital unit, community services, day
provision and whatever other elements there may be.
Where such a management system could be set up it
would allow proper planning of the transfer of money
and staff from one part of the service to another
and therefore aid the transition from hospital to
the community for patients and staff. The invisible
walls which are set up between management units at
present would at least be breached, allowing greater
communication and hence a greater likelihood of co-
ordination with social services, housing and the
voluntary sector.

Planning framework
The second step is to set up a planning framework.
If possible, statutory backing should be sought to
force all district health authorities to set up
joint planning teams at member and officer level for
mental health services in an area served by a single
large institution. That planning team should have
clear guidelines and timescales and its brief should
be simply to develop a comprehensive local service
in each district. Such joint planning teams should
include members of each health authority served by
the large institution, representatives of the local
authorities and voluntary organisations. The officer
level team could include representatives of housing
departments, housing associations, social service
departments and leisure departments as well as
voluntary organisations and regional health
authorities. Such a committee could be called a
single service or mental health service development
group. Regional health authorities have a vital role
to play in co-ordinating district health authorities
and in working with the DHSS Regional Social Work

Advisory Service to co-ordinate local authority
responses. Once regions have the right idea about
the sort of services required - and this is why we
must develop a blueprint for a comprehensive service
so that regional health authorities plan on the
basis of accepted principles - then regions are in a
strong position to encourage the development of
services and to find money. One way in which money
is being found at the present time is through what
is known as top-slicing of district health authority
budgets. Sadly, at present, that top-slicing does
not seem to be lowering some of the mountains we are
trying to climb and indeed, is only exacerbating the
other cuts in NHS budgets, such as the unfunded wage
award in 1982-3 and the so-called 0.5 per cent
efficiency saving demanded from district budgets in
the years from 1983-4 onwards.

Information
The third requirement will be to survey all patients
in long-stay provision to elicit their needs,
capabilities and potential, and to decide which
patients can be cared for in less institutional
environments. That does not mean that we are looking
only for those patients in existing hospitals who
can live without minimum support. We are saying that
those patients should not be in long-stay provision
and could be in ordinary housing with appropriate
support. Assessment of present long-stay patients
should be undertaken by staff from the relevant
hospital, with external moderation by a team of
skilled people. External criteria should be
established, following the principles listed above,
and assessments should be monitored critically
against those criteria. Determination of the
requirements of a community service will then draw
on the range of norms suggested by DHSS, modified by
assessment of the levels of care needed by patients
locally, and supplemented by information about
perceived needs of the local community from
statutory and voluntary agencies and consumer
groups. If necessary, special research should be
undertaken to establish the detailed needs for
special services or by particular categories of
clients.

Planning the service
Once these first three steps have been taken a start
can be made in planning the provision of the
service. The planning should include discussions
with all staff affected both in health authorities

and local authorities. Much current planning is
woolly and ill-considered and often does not involve
staff until the staff themselves become extremely
worried about their career progression or indeed
whether they are going to have a job at all in a
year or two. Trades Unions must be brought in at an
early stage on issues of remuneration. Retraining
and such matters as car allowances and mobility
provision to enable nursing staff to get out into
the community need to be considered. Staff should be
given the opportunity, at local level, to be
involved in the build-up of plans. Because,
traditionally, districts have not had a member level
forum, the health service seems to be unaware of the
need for accountability and to discuss issues with
representatives of the community. For any local
councillor who has had to work through the
democratic process, the undemocratic nature of
district health authorities comes as quite a shock.

Funding
The next step is, of course, to make best use of the
'Care in the Community' proposals, mentioned in many
chapters throughout this book. These involve
extending joint funding arrangements to 100 per cent
joint funding from health authorities to local
authorities for ten years with a three year
tapering; and to enable lump sum funding from health
authorities to local authorities for those patients
discharged from NHS care into that of the local
authority. None of these proposals brings any
significant additional money into the service and
additional cash should be made available. An
additional £50 million over and above existing
budgets is needed now, growing rapidly to £200
million per annum within five years. That would be
for England and Wales only. Even that is a small
amount of money, but central government and health
authorities must be made aware that if comprehensive
local mental health services are to be developed
additional money will be required to build up
community services before running down the large
hospitals. We know, for example, that taking a 1,000
bed mental illness hospital, it is unlikely that any
significant saving will be made until the number of
patients is reduced by at least 30 per cent, and no
real savings will be achieved until the number of
patients has been reduced by half. Health and local
authorities will be paying for two services in
tandem initially, with additional costs for planning
and development of the new services. Psychiatric

services must be fully community-oriented and have
sufficient facilities and appropriately trained
staff and managers before patients can be discharged
from the large mental illness hospitals.

Local authorities will have to accept that
earmarked funding will be given to provide services
for mentally ill and mentally handicapped people.
Such earmarked funding could come directly from
central government or from regional pools. But any
headway in service provision will have to be a two-
way process. As indicated at the beginning of this
chapter a 'bottom up' approach to planning the needs
of each district should be initiated. The basis for
planning should be defined locally and brought
together in an overall plan related to the needs of
individuals within the district. There will then be
some kind of 'top down' imposition of services
backed by appropriate funding from regional health
authorities, the Department of the Environment and
the DHSS.

Many local authorities will not like earmarked
funding but it seems the only way in which plans for
comprehensive services can be fulfilled within an
acceptable timescale. After all, 'community care'
started in the 1950s, and it is now over twenty
years since Enoch Powell made his famous 'water
towers' speech about closing the large hospitals.
Since then only one hospital has closed. In addition
to earmarked funding, without harming patient care,
large institution budgets should be squeezed in
order to force the transfer of patients. Experience
suggests that without some stick as well as carrot
professional staff will not make serious efforts to
move patients out of the long-stay wards into a
community setting.

Accountability
All of this requires a local forum for discussion
and accountability in the community. A forum should
involve professionals from NHS and local authority
services together with voluntary organisations. The
forum should make clear agreements as to the parts
of the service provided by different sections. Once
we have that agreement we can look at the aims and
objectives of the different parts of the service, we
can agree training requirements for the voluntary
sector and we can set up a grievance procedure to
ensure that problems are aired whether they occur in
the voluntary sector or the statutory sector. A
basic tenet of ths approach must be accountability
to the community and, as we have seen, this is not

something at which the health authorities excel.

Collaboration
There are significant ways in which local authorities, health authorities and the voluntary sector can work together. The voluntary sector simply cannot, and should not, take over major aspects of services. But the voluntary sector has a major role in bridging the gaps between health authorities and the community. The voluntary sector is sometimes able to get money which statutory services are unable to obtain and can, by this means, provide community services, particularly supported housing schemes, low-key day centres, self-help groups and sheltered employment schemes. Representatives of social services departments, leisure services and housing must all be involved in discussions. Health and housing are closely related, and it has always seemed a pity that they were separated in governmental terms.

Finally no one should fall into the trap of believing that 'community care' is a cheap option. It is not a cheap option, never has been and it should not be allowed to become one. On the other hand, community care is not necessarily any more expensive than the average costs for hospitals. Information collected within the Guys' Health District at the beginning of 1980 on mental handicap services showed that the cost of providing a full range of services for all the mentally handicapped people in the district was between £9,000 and £10,000 per annum: roughly the median cost, at that time, of provision in this country. The range of costs for hospitals is from £6,000 a year to around £16,000 a year per person. Community care is therefore no more expensive on average but is certainly not a cheap option.

We have, over the past 15 years, seen the discharge of patients into the community who were relatively able to cope because, perhaps, they should not have been in hospital in the first place or certainly not for such a long time. But we are now seeing a different population of patients being discharged who must be provided with continuing support in the community. I sympathise with those professional staff who are concerned that patients will be dumped in the community, but that is not what I am advocating. I do not wish to see patients dumped. I want to see properly funded comprehensive services and reports such as the Barclay Report (1982), presenting woolly, ill-considered proposals

for provision to the social work services are
worrying. Roger Hadley and Stephen Hatch (1981) have
rightly pointed to the fact that many clients are
cared for in the community by informal carers. For
example, nearly 70 per cent of elderly mentally
infirm people are cared for by informal carers in
ordinary houses. Hadley and Hatch go on to say that
informal carers should be given more support and the
logic of that cannot be faulted. However, it is a
significant leap of imagination to go from there to
suggest, as some commentators have, that all elderly
mentally infirm people should be cared for in the
community by informal carers. That is a nonsense.
Community care, in my view, is a humanising trend to
reintegrate people into community. It is not a
political rhetoric cutting the cost of services. De-
institutionalisation does not mean de-
professionalising the service, though we may well be
better able to make better use of volunteers and
better use of the community if we support those
volunteers and informal carers better. There will be
a need for a range of services for hospital
services, for clinics or self help groups for
prevention and a whole range of services locally.
With participation and collaboration between
voluntary services and the two main arms of the
statutory services - local authorities and health
authorities - we can build an effective
comprehensive local mental health service but it
does mean effective participation; it means tackling
issues such as confidentiality and it means
professional staff being open-minded about views
expressed from the community.

It is impossible in a single chapter such as
this to set out fully how one should implement a
comprehensive service. In any case each district is
different in its politics, its personalities and its
problems. This chapter has tried to suggest some
options for overcoming some of the problems. We may
not have turned the mountains into molehills but I
hope we can reach the point where we only push the
boulder once more up the hill and when we get it to
the top it will stay there and we can sit down and
rest, having generated a decent service. We owe it
to the consumers to provide them with the best
service we can.

REFERENCES

Barclay P M (Chairman) (1982). <u>Social Workers: Their Role and Tasks</u>. Bedford Square Press, London.
Black Report (1980). <u>Inequalities in Health</u>. DHSS.
Doyal L (1981). <u>Political Economy of Health</u>. Pluto Press, London.
Hadley R & Hatch S (1981). <u>Social Welfare and the Failure of the State</u>. Allen and Unwin, London.
Wolfensberger W (1972). <u>The Principle of Normalization in Human Services</u>. National Institute on Mental Retardation, Toronto. See also Lishman J (ed) (1981). <u>Normalisation</u>. Research Highlights No 2, Department of Social Work, University of Aberdeen.

Chapter Twenty-one

WHERE ARE WE NOW? SUMMARY AND CONCLUSIONS

Douglas Bennett

For many years there has been talk of transferring
the care of the mentally ill from mental hospitals
to other forms of provision in the community. Over
the years too, patients have been leaving mental
hospitals, whose populations have been reducing. At
the same time there has been a growth of
alternatives to care in institutions. Concomitantly
the ideas of comprehensive district psychiatric care
has developed. Progress inevitably has been slow,
and in meetings and in conferences discussion has
usually focussed on whether district psychiatric
services should, or could, substitute for mental
hospitals.

The conference, 'Cinderella No More', was
strikingly different since those questions were
rarely asked. Instead, as this book shows, speakers
and participants concentrated their attention on the
methods by which change could be brought about. This
does not mean, of course, that outside the
conference the forces of reaction, so dramatically
predicted by Enoch Powell in 1961, when he spoke of
'all the built-in tendencies to perpetuate the old',
have been dispelled. But it has meant that speakers
were free to explore new possibilities.

To date there has been much talk of moving
patients to the community and rather less about
moving staff and money. Too often these movements
have been seen as transferring segregated
psychiatric services in the mental hospital to
equally segregated psychiatric services in the wider
society. For many years ideas of hospital and
community provision have been polarised and there
has been little movement of ideas between the
different parts of the service. Yet, as this book
confirms, during the conference there was a movement
and a sharing of ideas among people with differing

outlooks   and   experiences.   Ideas   were   'de-
institutionalised'. There was an appreciation of the
fact that complex human problems cannot be solved by
one discipline or one agency alone. The needs of the
psychologically   stressed   or   the   psychiatrically
disordered were seen in terms of the everyday lives
of people in society rather than in the unreal life
of the psychotic patient in a mental hospital. Help
was no longer seen as being given by ward staff
alone. In this book it can be seen that author after
author emphasises the part played by family, friends
and neighbours with the supporting participation of
employers, housing and education authorities, the
general   health   services,   the   personal   social
services, social security and all kinds of voluntary
aid. The positive tone of all the chapters reflects
a willingness - even a determination - to overcome
the   difficulties   posed   by   different   trainings,
different jargons and different administrations.
There   is   an   unusual   endorsement   of   the
multidisciplinary,   multi-agency   approach: Edith
Morgan speaks of mutual respect and understanding
and Donald Dick draws attention to the spirit of the
highly effective working group. Bob Cawley also, in
his discussion of Lord Trefgarne's paper, emphasises
the need for co-operation between disciplines.
     Was this conference, then, a special occasion,
or did it truly signify a more general change of
outlook? Were the speakers and audience influenced
by   the   example   of   an   established   district
psychiatric service like that in the City and
Hackney District, or were they people who already
supported the move towards more local psychiatric
care? Does the changed outlook come from a
recognition that we are inevitably moving towards a
new situation? Some of those who did not attend this
conference may well feel, as they read this book,
that I have over-valued or attached too much
importance to the favourable attitudes expressed by
speakers and participants at the time. For them I
would say that it does not mean that there has been
any lack of realism. There has been no tendency to
underestimate the difficulties of effecting more
constructive combinations of hospital and community
services. Nor have the difficulties of sharing
insufficient resources been forgotten. There has,
perhaps, been too little emphasis on how the needs
of the very severely disabled and unfortunate
individuals who cause much distress not only to
their families and society but to hospital staff,
are to be catered for without recourse to mental

hospitals. There is not a great deal said about the nature of support, what it can and cannot do and how it should be organised. But these are not serious criticisms.

There is, of course, much to do. In the development of comprehensive psychiatric services we are, in the Churchillian phrase, not at the beginning of an end but approaching the end of a beginning. So the conference ended as it began, true to its title. Not only should there be no more fairy stories about institutionalised ogres in their mental hospitals or uncaring dragons roaming the community. There should be no more Cinderella psychiatric services in hospitals or outside. Instead, we should focus our attention and energies on making concerted efforts to develop effective, comprehensive psychiatric services in each district, responsive to the needs of their local communities.

BIBLIOGRAPHY

compiled by Geoffrey Baruch

Introduction

This bibliography reflects the developments which have taken place in the implementation of comprehensive district psychiatric services since 1976. Often, attention has been focussed on the inadequate progress made with such services, and this has led to a failure to appreciate the establishment of many community programmes. When compiling this bibliography, we were struck by the volume of literature describing programmes and projects, and since health and other professionals usually have little time to spend on writing, it seems highly likely that the schemes referred to here represent only the 'tip of the iceberg'. In other words, community mental health care has been implemented to a far greater extent than is often realised.

As the bibliography shows, there has also been a great deal of research during this period which has evaluated the effectiveness of different forms of care and examined their theoretical bases. Thus, for some districts at least, research and practice have combined to make community oriented mental health services a reality.

Needless to say, problems still remain. From the literature it appears that the main difficulties relate to the integration of elements of a service, to their financing, the role of the mental hospital in locally-based services, and the management of difficult and chronic patients.

All the items included in the bibliography are available in this country, either for reference at the King's Fund Centre library, 126 Albert Street, London NW1 7NF, or through other medical libraries. We have annotated entries where necessary to expand on the title or indicate particularly useful contents, and we have selected for inclusion only those books and articles which are relevant to psychiatric services in this country. The most useful way of organising the references seemed to be according to the various provisions within a community-based service. There are five sections: General Practice; Community Mental Health and Psychiatry; Psychiatric Units in District General Hospitals; Aftercare, Rehabilitation and Day Care; Residential Care and Occupation.

Contents

I	General Practice	216
II	Community Mental Health and Psychiatry	218
III	Psychiatric Units in District General Hospitals	229
IV	Aftercare, Rehabilitation and Day Care	233
V	Residential Care and Occupation	240

I GENERAL PRACTICE

ASHTON J R (1979)
The GP's role in psychiatric care.
Update, vol 18, no 3, pp 313-318.

BARSKY III A J (1980)
Defining psychiatry in primary care: origins, opportunities and obstacles.
Comprehensive Psychiatry, vol 21, no 3, pp 221-232.

BROOK A (1978)
An aspect of community mental health: consultative work with general practice
teams.
Health Trends, vol 10, pp 37-39.

BROOME A K & KAT B J B (1981)
Would more mental illness services help general practitioners manage their more
difficult patients?
Journal of the Royal College of General Practitioners, vol 31, no 226, 303-307

BURTON R H & FREELING P (1982)
How general practitioners manage depressive illness: a method of audit.
Journal of the Royal College of General Practitioners, vol 32, no 242, 558-561

CLARE A W (1979)
When patients are neurotic.
General Practitioner, June 15, p 55.
Investigates how GPs can deal with patients who have emotional problems which
do not warrant referral to a psychiatrist.

CLARE A W & CORNEY R H, Eds (1982)
Social Work and Primary Health Care.
Academic Press, London.
Collection of papers (mostly previously published). Topics covered include
social problems and ill health; the social worker and the primary care team;
social work intervention; evaluation of social work; and social and primary
care.

CLARE A W & LADER M, Eds (1982)
Psychiatry and General Practice.
Academic Press, London.
Collection of conference papers examining research into the nature and extent
of psychiatric illness. Areas discussed include epidemiology, treatment, and
the organisation of primary and psychiatric services.

CLARK D F (1979)
The clinical psychologist in primary care.
Social Science and Medicine, vol 13A, no 6, pp 707-713.

COLEMAN J V & PATRICK D L (1976)
Integrating mental health services into primary medical care.
Medical Care, vol 14, no 8, pp 654-661.
Argues in favour of integration of mental health providers and members of
primary care teams. Suggests that supportive services should be provided on a
continuing basis through patterned relationships, and that shared
responsibility for patient care between two professions provides built-in peer
review, and encourages inter-team consultation.

CORSER C M & RYCE S W (1977)
Community mental health care: a model on the primary care team.
British Medical Journal, vol 2, pp 936-938.
Describes a scheme, involving close contact between psychiatrists and general
practitioners, for providing mental health care. Anecdotal evidence suggests
that such a scheme can operate successfully.

DAVIDSON A F (1977)
Clinical psychology in general practice: a preliminary enquiry.
Bulletin of the British Psychological Society, vol 30, pp 337-338.

GOLDBERG D & HUXLEY P (1980)
Mental Illness in the Community
Tavistock, London.
An important book which reviews the present state of knowledge concerning the
factors that relate to four stages along the referral pathway: the decision to
consult, the detection of psychiatric illness by the doctor, referral to
psychiatric hospital outpatient services, and admission to inpatient care.
Includes results of a recent survey of 90 GPs which contains data on the
factors which determine doctors' sensitivity to emotional disturbance, and how
the personality of the doctor affects the awareness of disorder. Policy
implications are fully discussed.

KNIGHT L (1982)
GP - lynchpin for ex-mental patients.
Pulse, vol 42, no 13, p 34.
Outlines GP's role in providing aftercare in the wake of the Mental Health
(Amendment) Bill, which imposes this duty on authorities.

LAMBERT H (1979)
Problem behaviour in primary health care.
Journal of the Royal College of General Practitioners, vol 29, no 203, 331-335
Examines the role of primary health care team, especially non-medical members,
in helping patients with psycho-social problems.

MANN P (1979)
How a nurse taught doctors psychiatry.
General Practitioner, August 31, p 18.
Report of an eight-week experiment on how a community psychiatric nurse can
work in general practice.

McCORMACK M (1980)
Psychiatric help in the surgery.
General Practitioner, May 30, p 40.
Describes how there has been a huge drop in drug prescribing in an Oxfordshire
surgery since using a psychiatric counsellor.

McKECHNIE A, PHILIP A, & RAMAGE J G (1981)
Psychiatric services in primary care: specialised or not?
Journal of the Royal College of General Practitioners, vol 31, no 231, 611-614
Reports results of a study which confirms the findings of others in
demonstrating that there are tangible benefits from having a multi-disciplinary
specialist team working with psychiatric referrals in primary care.

McPHERSON I G & FELDMAN M P (1977)
A preliminary investigation of the role of the clinical psychologist in the
primary care setting.
Bulletin of the British Psychological Society, vol 30, pp 342-346.

MOTTRAM E M (1980)
The Sister's role in group therapy in a general practice.
Nursing Times, vol 76, no 6, pp 253-254.

SHEPHERD M (1980)
Mental Health as an integrant of primary medical care.
Journal of the Royal College of General Practitioners, vol 30, no 220, 657-664

TEMPERLY J (1978)
Psychotherapy in the setting of general practice.
British Journal of Medical Psychology, vol 51, pp 139-149.

THOMAS K B (1981)
Attitudes to psychological illness in general practice: a historical cycle
complete.
British Medical Journal, vol 283, pp 1157-1158.

TOUGH K, KINGERLEE P & ELLIOT P (1980)
Surgery-attached psychogeriatric nurses: an evaluation of psychiatric nurses in
the primary care team.
Journal of the Royal College of General Practitioners, vol 30, no 211, 83-85

WATSON J M & BARBER J H (1981)
Depressive illness in general practice: a pilot study.
Health Bulletin, vol 39, no 2, pp 122-116.
Shows how few patients receive counselling or are referred to a psychiatrist.
Findings based on 101 new episodes of depressive illness reported by nine GPs
in a three-month period.

WHITFIELD M J & WINTER R D (1980)
Psychiatry and general practice: results of a survey of Avon general
practitioners.
Journal of the Royal College of General Practitioners, vol 30, no 220, 682-686
Shows that considerable problems exist between GPs and psychiatrists over
the care of patients with mental illness.

WIJESINGHE B (1981)
The development of a community psychology service.
Journal of the Royal College of General Practitioners, vol 31, no 223, 113-115.
An important article showing how a primary mental health care service was
developed, having established the needs of GPs regarding the management of
patients with emotional problems.

WILLIAMS P (1982)
Psychiatry in general practice: the epidemiological approach.
Update, vol 24, no 3, pp 363-371.
Describes Goldberg and Huxley's model of psychiatric disorder in the community
and the relationship between different levels of care.

WILLIAMS P & CLARE A, Eds (1979)
Psychosocial Disorders in General Practice.
Academic Press, London.
Important collection of previously published papers with the editors
introducing sections on identification and patterns of psychosocial disorder;
factors altering risk for psychosocial disorder; management of psychosocial
disorder in general practice; the outcome of psychosocial disorder in general
practice; and future trends in research into primary care psychiatry.

WINTER R D & WHITFIELD M J (1980)
General Practitioners, counselling and psychotherapy.
Update, vol 20, no 6, pp 637-647.
According to the authors' survey, GPs believe that they should cope alone with
90 per cent of their patients with psychological problems, with the other 10
per cent being referred to the specialist psychiatric services.

II COMMUNITY MENTAL HEALTH AND PSYCHIATRY

ABRAHAMSON D & BRENNER D (1982)
Do long-stay psychiatric patients want to leave hospital?
Health Trends, vol 14, no 14, pp 95-97.
Surprisingly, many patients do. Argues that policy makers have failed to take
account of the wishes of patients in planning community services.

ALDER R (1978)
Allocation of resources.
Social Work Today, vol 9, no 43, p 21.
Discusses the problem of planning the allocation of resources for the mental
illness services between local authorities and the health service.

ANDERSON D (1981)
Why are people so reluctant to bring it to life?
Mindout, no 53, pp 18-21.
An excellent article which examines the gulf between policy and the failure to
make community care a reality.

ASHTON J R (1978)
Community care in psychiatry.
Community Care, vol 9, no 4, pp 211-215.
Argues in favour of more operational research to be conducted into mental
health services in order to establish the true application of community
psychiatry.

BABIGIAN H M (1977)
The impact of community mental health centres on the utilization of services.
Archives of General Psychiatry, vol 34, no 4, pp 385-394.

BARKER C (1977)
A community psychiatric service.
Nursing Times, vol 73, no 28, pp 1075-1079.
Reports on a research project to identify the organisation of patient care and
the role of the community psychiatric nurse in the District serviced by Powick
hospital, as it was run down and gradually replaced by community-based
facilities.

BARKER C (1981)
Into the community.
Health and Social Service Journal, vol XCI, no 4735, pp 315-318.
Examines the progress of the Worcester Development Project ten years after it
was launched.

BARNES R (1981)
The careless community.
Health and Social Service Journal, vol XCI, no 4762, p 1083.
Questions, from a social work view, the idea of community care, on the grounds
that the mentally ill can be even more isolated at home than in hospital due to
the fact that good neighbours simply do not exist for this group.

BENNETT D (1978)
Community Psychiatry.
British Journal of Psychiatry, vol 132, pp 209-220.
An extremely important and valuable article reviewing many aspects of community
psychiatry with some comparisons between the USA and Great Britain.

BENNETT D (1979)
De-institutionalisation in two cultures.
Millbank Memorial Fund Quarterly/Health and Society, vol 57, no 4, pp 516-532
Discusses historical process of de-institutionalisation in the USA and
Britain. Argues that 'de-institutionalisation and community care, having
similar starting points in both countries (USA and Great Britain), have
changed with time and the pressure of our different social and economic
systems'. (p 530).

BERGMAN K, FOSTER E M, JUSTICE A W, & MATHEWS V (1978)
Management of the demented elderly patient in the community.
British Journal of Psychiatry, vol 132, pp 441-449.
Argues that family support appears to be the most important factor determining
continuing life in the community, thus increased help to families from social
services is needed.

BEWLEY T H, BLAND M, MECHDEN D & WALCH E (1981)
New chronic patients.
British Medical Journal, vol 283, pp 1161-1164.
Study which shows that many new chronic patients were, in fact, old chronic
patients with intervals of community living. One third were likely to require
permanent care. Suggests that these findings provide no comfort for those who
believe that the present DHSS plans for the community-based mental health
services can ever be realised.

BISSONETTE R (1979)
The role of the clergy in community mental health service: a critical
assessment.
Psychiatry Quarterly, vol 51, no 4, pp 294-299.
The clergy appear to be both appropriate and available as a mental health
resource.

BRITISH ASSOCIATION OF SOCIAL WORKERS (1977)
Mental Health Crisis Services: A new philosophy.
Report of the evidence of the British Association of Social Workers on the
consultative document 'Review of the Mental Health Act 1959' and the White
Paper 'Better Services for the Mentally Ill'. Supports concentration of
services in the community as opposed to hospital-based services. Argues
that legislation should aim at relieving stress in the living situation
rather than moving the individual to hospital. Suggests the introduction
of a 24-hour emergency mental health programme.

BORN C (1981)
Research into rehabilitation and community care.
Mindout, no 50, pp 8-9.

BOSANQUET N (1977)
Services for the mentally ill.
Nursing Times vol 73, no 47, pp 1850-1855.
Looks at the extent of community-based provision - hostels, day care facilities
- and makes suggestions as to how services could be improved.

BOURAS N & BROUGH D I (1982)
The development of the mental health advice centre in Lewisham Health District.
Health Trends, vol 14, no 3, pp 65-69.
Describes the work of Handen Road Centre which aims to give a service
integrating primary health care with mental health professionals with easy
access for patients to psychiatric and psychological help.

BOWEN A (1979)
Some mental health premises.
Milbank Memorial Fund Quarterly, vol 57, no 4, pp 533-551.
An interesting paper which examines the idea of de-institutionalisation from a
historical perspective.

BRAFF J & LEFKOWITZ M M (1979)
Community Mental Health: what works for whom?
Psychiatric Quarterly, vol 51, no 2, pp 119-134.
A review of the literature aimed at identifying the type of services which are
effective for particular patient groups.

BROUGH D, COLLISON M, STIGLER M & BOWDEN R (1977)
Act now for mental health: multi-professional treatment for psychiatric cases.
Social Work Today, vol 8, no 40, pp 7-10.
Papers presented at conference 'Act now for Mental Health' which describe the
functioning of an integrated team meeting the needs of a district which has few
in-patient or day-patient facilities.

BUTTERWORTH C A & SKIDMORE D (1981)
Caring for the Mentally Ill in the Community.
Croom Helm, London.
A manual of treatment practice for those working with psychiatric patients in
the community. Views mental illness in terms of the effects on individual and
family.

BUTTERWORTH G (1983)
The community psychiatric nurse. A nurse for all seasons.
Primary Health Care, vol 1, no 2, p 9.

CARPENTER P J, DEL GAUDIO A C & MORGAN G R (1979)
Dropouts and terminators from a community mental health centre: their use of
other psychiatric services.
Psychiatric Quarterly, vol 51, no 4, pp 271-279.

CHRISTIE-BROWN J R W, EBRINGER L & FREEDMAN L S (1977)
A survey of a long-stay psychiatric population: implications for community
services.
Psychological Medicine, vol 7, pp 113-126.
Survey of 220 long-stay patients with assessment of accommodation and
employment needs. Results showed need for long-stay or permanent accommodation.
Careful discussion of validity of research methods.

CAMPBELL C (1983)
Community psychiatry: calm amid the storm.
Nursing Mirror, vol 156, no 5, pp 26-29.
Describes the work of a community psychiatric nurse in an inner London borough.

CAMPBELL W, DILLON A & DOW I (1983)
Management: a case for new training.
Nursing Mirror, vol 156, no 3, pp 42-40.
Examines the work of the community psychiatric nurse and argues the need for a
better definition of the CPN's task and a formal training programme.

CONWAY-NICHOLLS K & ELLIOT A (1982)
North Camden Community Psychiatric Nursing Service.
British Medical Journal, vol 285, no 6345, pp 859-861.

DARTFORD AND GRAVESHAM HEALTH DISTRICT (1980)
New approaches to the further development of community services for the
mentally ill.
Report of a seminar, Dartford and Gravesham HD, held prior to setting up a
local crisis intervention service.

DEAR M, CLARK G & CLARK S (1979)
Economic cycles and mental health care policy: an examination of the
macro-context for social service planning.
Social Science and Medicine, vol 13C, pp 43-53.
Demonstrates the links between the general state of the economy and mental
health care policy. Clear relationships are shown between the rates of
unemployment and inflation and the levels of admissions, discharge patients on
the books, vacancy rate and number of available beds in the one hospital
studied intensively.

DHSS (1979)
United Kingdom paper on Mental Health Policy Formulation submitted to
the World Health Organisation, July.
A summary of the state of play in the development of community mental
health services, and objectives for future policy.

DHSS (1981)
Homes and Hostels for the Mentally Ill and Mentally Handicapped. 1976 - 1980
DHSS, Personal Social Services, Local Authority Statistics.

DHSS (1983)
Mental Illness: Policies for prevention, treatment, rehabilitation and care.
A brief but comprehensive note on policies advocated by DHSS in various
circulars and advice notes.

DOWRICK C, MARKWICK M, MARTIN S & SMITH L (1980)
The Worcester experiment.
Social Work Today, vol 11, no 23, pp 10-15.
Four social workers involved in this project, which was designed to put into
practice the concept of community care embodied in the 'Better Services for the
Mentally Ill' analyse the experiment and its implications for the mental health
service generally.

EARLY D F & NICHOLAS M (1981)
Two decades of change: Glenside Hospital population surveys, 1960 to 1980.
British Medical Journal, vol 282, pp 1446-1449.
Although the patient population continues to be decreased, there is still an
accumulation of long-stay patients, mainly for non-medical reasons. Argues that
these patients remain in hospital because of a failure to provide community

facilities and suggests that the NHS should be enabled to extend their hospital
services into 'nursing homes' in the community.

EBRINGER L & CHRISTIE-BROWN J R W (1980)
Social deprivation amongst short-stay psychiatric patients.
British Journal of Psychiatry, vol 136, pp 46-52.
Findings which show hospitalisation contributes to social deprivation.

EURO REPORTS AND STUDIES 25 (1980)
Changing patterns in mental health care.
World Health Organisation.
Report discusses emerging trends in mental health care; planned innovations in
Italy, West Germany, Sweden and the USSR; and changing patterns of care for
sub-groups and special problems.

FENTON F R, TESSIER L, STRUENING E L, SMITH F A & BENOIT C (1982)
Home and Hospital Psychiatric Treatment.
Croom Helm, London.
A comparison of two treatment locations.

FINK P J & OKEN D (1976)
The role of psychiatry as a primary care speciality.
Archives of General Psychiatry, vol 33, no 8, pp 998-1003.

FOLKINS C & SPENSLEY J (1977)
Peer rating by a community mental health team: a positive approach to
accountability.
American Journal of Orthopsychiatry, vol 47, no 2, pp 331-335.

FOLKINS C, WEISELBERG N, & SPENSLEY J (1981)
Discipline stereotyping and evaluative attitudes amongst community mental
health staff.
American Journal of Orthopsychiatry, vol 51, no 1, pp 140-148.

FRANK R (1981)
Cost-benefit analysis for mental health services: a review of the literature.
Administration in Mental Health, vol 8, no 3, pp 161-176.

FREEMAN H, CHEADLE A J & KORER J R (1979)
A method for monitoring the treatment of schizophrenics in the community.
British Journal of Psychiatry, vol 134, pp 412-416.

GIBBON M (1980)
Psychiatry for the asking.
World Medicine, vol 15, no 10, pp 66-67.
Reports on a centre in Sussex designed to make psychiatric help available more
easily and informally than hospital services. Based on US model of psychiatric
advice clinics.

GLAZER W, SHOLOMKAS D, WILLIAMS D & WEISSMAN M (1982)
Chronic schizophrenics in the community: are they able to report their social
adjustment?
American Journal of Orthopsychiatry, vol 52, no 1, pp 166-171.
Argues that de-institutionalisation of schizophrenic patients makes it
imperative that a reliable and valid method of assessing social adjustment is
developed. This study focusses on data obtained from the administration of the
Social Adjustment Scale II.

GOOD PRACTICES IN MENTAL HEALTH
(International Hospital Federation) GPMH Information Service: 67 Kentish Town
Road, London NW1 8NY.
This project was started by the IHF in 1977. It promotes and publicises local
'Good Practices' studies which include local schemes which have been found to
work effectively a provide a useful service to mentally ill people. By the end
of 1981 twenty-two local studies had been produced from districts all over the
country. Leaflet, lists and information notes available from the project.

HEPTINSTALL D (1980)
Mentally ill: can we make the community care?
Community Care, no 306, pp 36-37.
Examines the problems of expanding community provision for mental illness.

HILL, PROFESSOR SIR DENNIS (1980)
Progress but in slow tempo.
Health and Social Service Journal, vol LXXXX, no 4701, pp 904-906.
Traces the advances made since 1930 and poses the question: how far have we
come since then?

HORNBLOW A R & SLOANE H R (1980)
Evaluating the effectiveness of a telephone counselling service.
British Journal of Psychiatry, vol 137, pp 377-388.

IN PRACTICE (1980)
Services for mental illness.
General Practitioner, November 14th, pp 31-48.
An edition devoted to mental health provision, including psychiatric units,
care for the elderly, alcoholism, retardation, child services and the role of
the GP.

JANSEN E (1980)
The Therapeutic Community outside the Hospital.
Croom Helm, London.
The contributors examine the role of the therapeutic community, both from a
professional and a policy-making perspective, and seek to identify the
particular contribution which the therapeutic community is able to make in
order to promote their full scale development as part of mental health
services.

JONES K (1977)
The wrong target in mental health.
New Society, vol 39, pp 438-440.
Attacks the civil liberties approach to solving mental illness problems in
favour of one which strives to implement an integrated service.

JOWELL T (1980)
Progressive Psychiatry under threat.
CHC News, no 58, p 11.
Examines the impact of cuts in local mental illness services.

KIRK S (1976)
Effectiveness of community services for discharged mental patients.
American Journal of Orthopsychiatry, vol 46, no 4, pp 646-659.
This study of 579 state hospital patients charts the pattern of their care in
the community in the two to three years following discharge from hospital. It
examines the relationship of aftercare services to readmission rates. Findings
suggest that among the most chronic patients a substantial number of aftercare
visits may be reflected in lower hospital readmission rates.

KNIGHT L (1977)
Still the Cinderella.
Community Care, no 156, pp 47-48.
Discusses the growing gap between mental health policy over the past twenty
years and its implementation.

LAMB R H & GOERTZEL V (1977)
The long-term patient in the era of community treatment.
Archives of General Psychiatry, vol 34, no 6, pp 679-682.
A study which examines the lives of a group of long-term disabled patients
living in the community and not usually encompassed by post-hospital follow-up
studies.

LAMB R H (1979)
The new asylums in the community.
Archives of General Psychiatry, vol 36, no 2, pp 129-134.
Argues that board-and-care homes for psychiatric patients offer them asylum

from life's pressures, a degree of structure and some treatment, especially the supervision of medication. For many long-term patients these homes have taken over the function of the state hospitals.

THE LANCET (1978)
Commentary from Westminster: 'Care of the Mentally Ill'.
The Lancet, vol 1, pp 1371-1372.
Reports Tory plan for promoting mental health care when Conservatives return to power.

LEACH J & WING J K (1978)
The effectiveness of a service for helping destitute men.
British Journal of Psychiatry, vol 133, pp 481-492.

LEUTZ W N (1976)
The informal community caregiver: a link between the health care system and local residents.
American Journal of Orthopsychiatry, vol 46, no 4, pp 678-688.
A study which shows that community health services would benefit from having informal caregivers.

LEVINE M (1981)
The History and Politics of Community Mental Health (USA).
OUP, New York.

LINN M W, CAFFREY E, KLETT C J & HOGARTY G (1977)
Hospital versus community (foster) care for psychiatric patients.
Archives of General Psychiatry, vol 34, no 1, pp 78-83.
Study which suggests that foster care is superior to hospitalisation for patients who cannot return to their own homes.

MANCHESTER J (1983)
A Framework for Planning.
Nursing Mirror, vol 156, no 15, pp 34-36.
Shows how the introduction of the nursing process into a community psychiatric nursing setting in Graylingwell Hospital, Sussex, produced a remarkable improvement in the service.

MANGEN S P & GRIFFITH J H (1982)
Patient satisfaction with community psychiatric nursing: a prospective controlled study.
Journal of Advanced Nursing, vol 7, no 5, pp 477-482.

MANGEN S P & GRIFFITH J H (1982)
Community psychiatric nursing services in Britain: the need for policy and planning.
International Journal of Nursing Studies, vol 19, no 3, pp 157-166.

MARSTAL H B (1980)
Developing comprehensive mental health services.
World Hospitals, vol 16, no 4, pp 36-38.

MEACHER M (1979)
New Methods of Mental Health Care.
Pergamon, London.
Although not comprehensive in its coverage, this book contains contributions which discuss many important developments in the aftercare of patients and the prevention of mental disturbance. Includes experimental preventive services which have been systematically evaluated, new techniques for care of the elderly confused, new approaches by different caring groups and the problems of specific patient populations.

THE MENTAL HEALTH FOUNDATION (1978)
A selection of pioneering community mental health services supported by the MHF.
Mental Health Foundation, London.

Bibliography   225

MENTAL HEALTH TRUST AND RESEARCH FUND (1976)
Pioneering Community Mental Health Services supported by the MHT & RF in
1974/5.
Projects funded by MHT & RF were designed to fill gaps in community-based
services.

MIND (1976)
MIND report: Effective community care and the mentally ill.
Discusses back-up resources for GPs, hostel staff and others caring for the
mentally ill in the community.

MIND (1977)
Evidence to the Royal Commission on the NHS with regard to services
for mentally ill people.
Makes a strong plea for a full range of community psychiatric services.

MIND (1978)
A new deal for mental patients.
Further evidence to the Royal Commission on the NHS.

MIND (1979)
Prevention in Mental Health.
MIND Annual Conference proceedings, 1979.
Topics covered include mental health in the community, mental health in the
workplace, women and children, mental health aspects of antenatal, intranatal
and postnatal care.

MIND (1980)
Alternatives to Mental Hospitals.
Report of a European workshop, Parts 1 & 2.
A fascinating series of papers presented by leading European figures, in favour
of community methods of mental health care. Topics covered include sheltered
accommodation, day care, the role of volunteers, strategic issues in the move
away from mental hospitals, crisis intervention, district psychiatric
rehabilitation.

MIND (1982)
Projects run by local associations, January 1982.
A geographical run-down of various schemes for the mentally ill, including
group homes, hostels and half-way houses, flatlets, bedsits, sheltered
accommodation, social clubs and day centres.

MIND Information Bulletin (Dec 1981/Jan 1982)
Community Mental Health Service Report on LINK.
Scheme run by Glasgow Association for Mental Health which serves as a community
resource centre.

MORGAN E (1978)
Community involvement in mental health (London).
World Hospitals, vol 14, p 16.
Shows how ordinary people can complement the services of their communities in
important and distinctive ways.

MORGAN E (1980)
Good practices in mental health.
World Hospitals, vol 16, pp 10-14.
Account of the GPMH project since 1977.

MORLEY D (1980)
Under One Roof.
Castle Street Circular, no 120, pp 4-6.
New counselling and resource centre in Livepool.

MORRIS P (1980)
Working for mental health in Sheffield.
Mindout, no 38, p 24.
The work and problems of the Lawton Tonge Centre, designed to meet variable
needs of clients.

MURPHY E (1983)
Old age and depression in the East End of London.
New Age, no 21, pp 22-24

NURSING TIMES (1977)
The Worcester Development Project.
Nursing Times, vol 73, no 28.
Various articles describing how a system of care based on mental hospitals was
replaced by a fully integrated community psychiatric service.

OLDHAM A J & GAIND R C (1977)
Community psychiatry in a London borough; an eleven year analysis of a
socio-medical service for psychiatric illness.
British Journal of Psychiatry, vol 130, pp 355-364:

OZARIN L D & SHARFSTEIN S S (1978)
The aftermath of de-institutionalisation: problems and solutions.
Psychiatric Quarterly, vol 50, no 2, pp 128-132.

PAVITT B (1981)
Building bridges for better services.
Health and Social Service Journal, vol XCI, no 4746, pp 677-678.
Reports on a project which successfully uses volunteers in mental health
services.

PAYKEL E S, MANGEN S P, GRIFFITH J H & BURNS T P (1982)
Community psychiatric nursing for neurotic patients: a controlled trial.
British Journal of Psychiatry, vol 140, pp 573-581.
Shows that the care of neurotic patients by community psychiatric nurses is
effective and efficient and a valuable mode of deployment within the
psychiatric team.

PAYNE M (1979)
Social bridging.
Health and Social Service Journal, vol LXXXIX, no 4672, p 1002.
Describes a new journal 'Dovetail' launched in Bristol and directed towards
encouraging the community to participate in mental health problems.

POLACK P R & KIRBY M W (1976)
A model to replace psychiatric hospitals.
Journal of Nervous and Mental Disease, vol 162, no 1, pp 13-22.
An interesting study showing that community treatment is more effective than
psychiatric hospitalisation.

POSTLEWATE J (1979)
Informality helps the disturbed mind.
Pulse, vol 39, no 21, p 18.
The walk-in service at Lewisham's mental health centre.

PRITLOVE J (1978)
What future for the mentally ill?
Community Care, no 208, pp 20-22.
Traces the theory and practice of community care for the mentally ill since the
1959 Mental Health Act, and looks to the future.

PSYCHIATRIC QUARTERLY (1978)
An issue devoted to community services for the mentally ill.
Psychiatric Quarterly, vol 50, no 4.
Topics include the establishment of services, community residences, services
which have been successful and those which have failed, rehabilitation.

PSYCHIATRIC QUARTERLY (1980)
An issue devoted to community mental health.
Psychiatric Quarterly, vol 52, no 1.
Topics include the delivery of community mental health services in New York
State and the planning and evaluation of community mental health programmes.

RATNA L (1982)
Crisis intervention in psychogeriatrics.
British Journal of Psychiatry, vol 141, September, pp 296-301.
A study of a community-oriented psychogeriatric service in North London.

THE RICHMOND FELLOWSHIP (1983)
Mental Health and the Community.
Richmond Fellowship Press, London.
A detailed enquiry into mental health services. Invaluable report, with
comprehensive coverage of community care, from theoretical base to
implementation. Useful section on financial implications.

ROLLIN H (1977)
Editorial: Deinstitutionalisation and the community: fact and theory.
Psychological Medicine, vol 7, pp 181-184.
Full discussion of the extent to which implications of the 1959 Mental Health
Act and subsequent policy objectives have been fulfilled, and the extent to
which the aims of care in the community remain latent.

ROWBOTTOM R & HEY A (1978)
Organisation of services for the mentally ill.
Brunel Institute of Organisation and Social Studies.
Draws on research into the problems of developing a domiciliary mental health
service.

RYAN J (1980)
Life outside the institutions.
Mindout, no 40, p 11.
Research into lives of short-stay patients with chronic or long-term illness.

SCHMIDT L J, REINHARDT A M, KANE R L & OLSEN D D (1977)
The mentally ill in nursing homes.
Archives of General Psychiatry, vol 34, no 6, pp 687-691.
A study which shows that patients in this community setting experienced an
increase in prescribed psycho-active medication and a decrease in activity. The
authors question the reliance on nursing homes for the care of psychiatric
patients.

SCOTT R D & SECCOMBE P (1976)
Community Psychiatry - setting up a service on a shoe-string.
Mindout, no 17, pp 5-7.
The implementation of a crisis intervention service at Napsbury Hospital using
no extra money or manpower. An important paper since it discusses the
resistance of the community to such intervention.

SCOTT R D (1980)
A family oriented psychiatric service in the London Borough of Barnet.
Health Trends, vol 12, no 3, pp 65-68.
Brings up to date Scott's own particular approach to community mental health
care, the basic orientation being family psychiatry and the family doctor.

SEGAL S P & AVIRAM U (1978)
The mentally ill in community-based sheltered care: a study of community care
and social integration.
John Willey & Sons, New York.

SHEPHERD G C (1981)
Don't forget the mentally disabled.
Mindout, no 45, pp 12-14.

STEIN L I & TEST M A (1980)
Alternative to Mental Hospital Treatment.
Archives of General Psychiatry, vol 37, pp 392-397.
Conceptual model for community-based support programme for chronically disabled
psychiatric patients. When put into practice and compared with conventional
support the need for hospitalisation was reduced. When special support was
withdrawn patients relapsed into patterns of conventional care, and improvement
was not maintained.

TORBAY HEALTH AUTHORITY & SOUTH DEVON SOCIAL SERVICES (1983)
Community Mental Health Centres: the Way Forward.
Paper proposing the development of CHMC network in South Devon.

TOWELL D (1978)
Developing   services   based   on   large   institutions: some   organisational
requirements.
Health Services Manpower Review, vol 4, no 2, pp 3-6.
Discusses the problems involved in the long transition from institutional based
care   to community systems. Argues   that   within   the options created by the
resources which   can be made available there is much that appropriate
organisation and management can do to facilitate, foster and support the
development of better services.

TRIMBOS E (1978)
Developments   in   intra-mural   and   extra-mural   alternatives   to   the   mental
hospital.
World Hospitals, vol 16, no 4, pp 22-25.
A review of international developments in community psychiatry.

WALKEY F H, GREEN D E, & TAYLOR A J W (1981)
Community attitudes to mental health: a comparative study.
Social Science and Medicine, vol 15E, pp 139-144.
A study which demonstrates the reluctance of local communities to play a major
role in the treatment and rehabilitation of the mentally ill.

WERTHEIMER A (1979)
Cutting the lifeline to mental health.
Mindout, no 35, pp 17-19.
Considers the effects of expenditure cuts on mental health services.

WHITEHEAD T (1977)
Localising mental health care.
Mindout, no 24, pp 12-14.
Notes that progess towards community care and the phasing out of mental
hospitals has been piecemeal. Suggests that semi-autonomous units could be
created in mental hospitals staffed by multi-disciplinary teams serving
particular geographical areas.

WHO (1979)
Changing patterns in mental health care in Europe.
WHO Chronicle, vol 33, no 5, pp 180-182.
Notes the failure of many regions in running down their mental hospitals, but
acknowledges the establishment of many experimental community mental health
programmes in different parts of Europe. Examines some criteria by which the
success of individual projects can be judged, and some of the steps that can
contribute to more effective mental health care in a community setting.

WILLIAMS P & CLARE A (1981)
Changing patterns of psychiatric care.
British Medical Journal, vol 282, pp 375-377.
Examines the issue of whether psychiatric care since the end of the 1960s has
shifted from general practice to the specialist psychiatric services.

WING J K (1981)
From institutional to community care.
Psychiatric Quarterly, vol 53, no 2, pp 140-151.
A keynote address presented at the second annual Hyman M Forstenzer symposium,
Albany, New York, 1980. The paper is concerned mainly with the group of
patients who used to accumulate in the mental hospitals - those referred with
symptoms of schizophrenia, paranoid psychosis or manic-depressive illness. It
examines the developments in British services and gives an extremely concise
and informative review of the issues.

WING J K (Ed) (1982)
Long-term Community Care: Experience in a London Borough.
Psychological Medicine, Monograph Supplement No 2.
An important study comprising a survey of long-term users of the community
psychiatric services in Camberwell, and an evaluative study of a hostel-ward
for 'new' long-stay patients.

WING J K, BEBBINGTON P & ROBINS L N (1981)
What is a case? The problem of definition in psychiatric community surveys.
Grant, McIntyre, London.
The contributors to this book examine the theoretical and methodological issues
involved in measuring psychiatric disorder.

WING J K & OLSEN R (1979)
Community Care for the Mentally Disabled.
Oxford University Press, Oxford.

YOUNG M (1977)
Treating the long-term mentally ill.
Social Work Today, vol 9, no 10, pp 11-12.
Argues that social workers are needed by long-term mentally ill, and have a
definite role to play in improving the quality of life in both field and
residential settings.

III PSYCHIATRIC UNITS IN DISTRICT GENERAL HOSPITALS

BALLINGER B R, CAMERON L, MUNRO A & SCOTT J C (1981)
Inter-district comparison of geriatric psychiatry services.
Health Bulletin, vol 39, no 4, pp 228-235.

BARUCH G F & TREACHER A (1978)
Treating the mentally ill.
New Society, vol 44, pp 125-127.
On the basis of a study of a psychiatric unit, argues that change from mental
hospital may be meaningless if the original methods of operation and
organisation are transferred to a new treatment setting.

BARUCH G F & TREACHER A (1978)
Psychiatry Observed.
Routledge and Kegan Paul, London.
A controversial book which contains two chapters on the evolution of
psychiatric units in general hospitals.

BOTT E (1976)
Hospital and Society.
British Journal of Medical Psychology, vol 49, pp 97-140.
A substantial and interesting paper which examines the social control functions
of mental hospitals and relates these to definitions of mental illness within
society.

BOWMAN M J & STURGEON D A (1977)
A clinic within a general hospital for the assessment of urgent psychiatric
problems.
The Lancet, vol II, pp 1067-1068.

BRITISH MEDICAL JOURNAL, Editorial (1976)
Asylums are still needed.
British Medical Journal, vol 1, pp 111-112.

BROOKS P & WALTON H J (1981)
Liaison psychiatry in Scotland.
Health Bulletin, vol 39, no 4, pp 218-227.
Discusses the role of liaison psychiatry in general hospitals in Scotland -
i.e. the provision of psychiatric care to patients and advice to professional
staff within the general, or 'non-psychiatric' environment.

CAMPBELL W (1978)
Problems of the small unit.
Health and Social Service Journal, vol LXXXVIII, no 4580, p 218.
Focusses on problems of coping with violent, elderly and long-stay patients in
psychiatric units.

COPAS J B, FREEMAN-BROWNE D L & ROBIN A A (1977)
Treatment settings in psychiatry. The use of hospital services: long term
follow up.
British Journal of Psychiatry, vol 130, pp 365-369.
A study which finds little difference in the treatment careers of patients
whose first admission was either in a mental hospital or in a general hospital
psychiatric unit.

FEINMAN J (1979)
An example of what was once planned to replace the old mental hospitals.
Medical News, vol 11, no 26, p 7.
Describes the newly-opened psychiatric unit at Southampton General Hospital,
one of the last 'custom-built' psychiatric hospital.

FLOWERS J & SAUNDERS E (1980)
Long-term psychiatric patients serviced by the psychiatric unit at Queen
Elizabeth II Hospital, Welwyn Garden City.
Social Services Research Group Journal, vol 136, pp 205-215.
Provides information, based on a detailed survey, about services available for
patients who suffer from chronic or long-term mental illness in an area which
has no access to traditional long-stay beds. Looks at the support needs of
patients in this category.

GASPAR D (1980)
Hollymoor Hospital Dementia Service.
The Lancet, vol 1, pp 1402-1405.
Shows how prompt domiciliary assessment, neurological treatment and community
help arranged by the dementia service enabled more than a third of patients
referred to be managed at home.

GLICK I D, HARGREAVES W A, DRUES J & SHOWSTACK J A (1976)
Short versus long hospitalization: a prospective controlled study. IV: one-year
follow-up results for schizophrenic patients.
American Journal of Psychiatry, vol 133, no 5, pp 509-514.
Finds that a long-term approach is more beneficial than a short-term one for
schizophrenic patients.

GLICK I D, HARGREAVES W A, DRUES J & SHOWSTACK J A (1976)
Short versus long hospitalization: a prospective controlled study. V: one year
follow-up results for non-schizophrenic patients.
American Journal of Psychiatry, vol 133, no 5, pp 515-517.
Results show few differences resulting from length of hospitalization for
this group of patients.

GREENHILL M H (1979)
Psychiatric units in general hospitals: 1979.
Hospital and Community Psychiatry, vol 30, no 3, pp 169-182.
Presents an overview of psychiatric units in general hospitals. Summarises
evaluative studies and proposes further ones aimed at assessing the effects of
short-term treatment.

GRIMES J A (1978)
The probability of admission to a mental hospital or unit.
Health Trends, vol 10, no 1, pp 13-14.

HERZ M I, ENDICOTT J & SPITZER R L (1977)
Brief Hospitalization: a two year follow-up.
American Journal of Psychiatry, vol 134, no 5, pp 502-507.
Results confirm that brief hospitalization is preferable to longer-term for
most patients.

HENDLER N, WISE T N & LUCAS M J (1979)
The expanded role of the psychiatric liaison nurse.
Psychiatric Quarterly, vol 51, no 2, pp 135-143.

HIRSCH S R, PLATT S, KNIGHTS A & WEYMAN A (1979)
Shortening hospital stay for psychiatric care: effect on patients and their
families.
British Medical Journal, vol II, pp 442-446.
Findings show the value of shortening hospital stay with the proviso that day
care facilities are increased to give continuing treatment and aftercare.

HOLMES W & SOLOMON P (1980)
Criteria used in first admissions and readmissions to psychiatric hospitals.
Social Science and Medicine, vol 14A, no 1, pp 55-59.

THE HOSPITAL AND SOCIAL SERVICES REVIEW (1976)
New psychiatric unit at the Whittington Hospital.
The Hospital and Social Services Review, vol 72, no 9, pp 313-314.

HOWAT J (1979)
Nottingham and the Hospital Plan: A follow-up study of long-stay inpatients.
British Journal of Psychiatry, vol 135, pp 42-51.
A fifteen-year attrition study of 1960 long-stay inpatients in Nottingham's
psychiatric hospitals shows a high rate of discharge, especially for males. The
reasons for these findings and some implications are discussed.

JEEVENDRAPILLAI V & CAMPBELL W (1979)
A study of new long-stay patients in a psychiatric unit : identifying the
dependency of these patients in a small psychiatric unit.
Nursing Times, vol 75, no 15, pp 633-637.

KEILL S L (1980)
Psychiatric care: a new role for hospitals.
Hospitals, vol 54, no 19, pp 67-70.
Argues that psychiatric units should play a key role in the provision of
services because of their unique situation regarding accessibility, image and
range of resources.

KENNEDY P & HIRD F (1980)
Description and evaluation of a short-stay admission ward.
British Journal of Psychiatry, vol 136, pp 205-215.
Describes a number of benefits which arise because of short-term admissions.

THE LANCET (1979)
Psychiatric illness among medical patients.
The Lancet, vol 1, no 8114, pp 478-479.
Findings about the extent of psychiatric illness among medical patients
provides support for psychiatric units situated in general hospitals.

LAUER J W (1977)
Some demographic characteristics of a psychiatric inpatient unit in an urban
general hospital.
Illinois Medical Journal, vol 152, no 3, pp 212-218.

LIPOWSKI Z J (1981)
Liaison psychiatry, liaison nursing and behavioural medicine.
Comprehensive Psychiatry, vol 22, no 6, pp 554-561.
Discusses the role of liaison psychiatry - the area of psychiatry which is
concerned with the diagnosis, treatment, study and prevention of psychiatric
morbidity in the physically ill.

LLOYD G C (1980)
Whence and whither 'liaison' psychiatry?
Psychological Medicine, vol 10, pp 11-14.

LOMAS G (1979)
Long-term Mental Illness in Hackney.
Community Psychiatry Research Unit, Working Note No. 1.
Describes the characteristics of a one-year cohort of long-term in and out
patients in a general hospital psychiatric unit and assesses their
accommodation and occupation needs.

MAHADEVAN S & FORSTER D P (1982)
Psychiatric units in general hospitals and traditional mental hospitals: some
recent evidence.
British Journal of Psychiatry, vol 140, pp 160-165.
Argues that the operational policies practiced by psychiatrists are more
important than the structure of the system, and suggests that it is important
to establish policies for a variety or organisational structures.

McPHAIL N I (1978)
Behavioural disturbances in a general hospital psychiatric unit.
Health Bulletin, vol 36, no 2, pp 79-88.
Reflects the concern of psychiatrists about the ability of psychiatric units to
contain 'difficult' behaviour. Argues that such behaviour can be managed
satisfactorily.

MEDICAL NEWS (1979)
No more psychiatric units to be built?
Medical News, vol 11, no 26, p 2.
Reports government decision to halt the building of psychiatric units.

PUBLIC HEALTH (1981)
Mental illness hospitals: high goals, wrong objectives.
Public Health, vol 95, no 3, pp 127-128
An editorial which suggests that the role of the mental hospital requires
re-consideration, given the failure to achieve a service based on psychiatric
units in district general hospitals.

PULLEN I (1980)
Admission rate of old people to Scottish psychiatric units.
British Medical Journal, vol 281, p 843.

ROBIN A A, COPAS J B & FREEMAN-BROWNE D L (1979)
Treatment settings in psychiatry: long-term family and social findings.
British Journal of Psychiatry, vol 135, pp 35-41.
A study which shows that treatment in a psychiatric unit, as distinct from a
psychiatric hospital, held the benefits in the long-term (5 - 8 years after
admission) as far as the patient's mental and behavioural status and
employment, and the family's burdens, health needs and attitudes were
concerned.

ROLLIN A (1976)
Are mental hospitals really necessary?
Public Health, vol 90, no 2, pp 49-52.
Questions the wisdom of closing down mental hospitals.

ROONEY P & MATTHEWS R (1982)
Worcester Development Project Psychiatric Provision - where do we go from
here?
Mental Health Buildings Evaluation Pamphlet 3.
DHSS Works Group, London.

ROSS T (1977)
Deaf unit, Whittington Hospital: a psychiatric unit for the deaf.
Nursing Mirror, 24 November, pp 20-22.

SANSOM-FISHER R W, DESMOND POOLE A & THOMSON V (1979)
Behaviour patterns within a general hospital psychiatry unit: an observational
study.
Behaviour Research and Therapy, vol 17, pp 317-332.
Revealing study which shows that staff spent the majority of their time in the

unit engaged in interaction with their peers or on their own work, with little time being spent with patients. Patients spent half their time in solitary activities, and when they were observed interacting with others it was usually with other patients.

SCHULMAN K & ARIE T (1978)
Fall in admissions of old people to psychiatric units.
British Medical Journal, vol 1, pp 156-158.
Examines the reasons for old people failing to obtain inpatient care.

SCHWAB P J (1977)
The evolution of a general hospital psychiatric unit.
Current Psychiatric Therapies, vol 17, pp 301-308.
Records the development of a unit according to the changes in the types of treatment models used over a period of twenty years.

SYKES P (1976)
Integrated psychiatric care.
Medical Record, vol 17, no 2, pp 125-132.
WATTS C C (1977)
In praise of units.
Health and Social Service Journal, vol LXXXVII, p 1378.

WHITEHEAD T (1976)
A plan for psychiatric hospitals.
Health and Social Service Journal, vol LXXXVI, p 981.

WHITEHEAD T (1981)
A single-ward approach to the elderly mentally ill.
Health Trends, vol 13, no 4, pp 99-100.
Describes a service for the elderly mentally ill which is based in a general hospital complex and combines a heavy community commitment with the use of two all-purpose wards and two associated day hospitals.

WHITEHEAD T (1983)
Mental infirmity - the Cottage Hospital approach.
Geriatric Medicine, vol 13, no 2, pp 99-103.
Describes the service offered in Brighton, where patients are supported at home if at all possible, with adequate day hospital facilities backed-up by a small inpatient unit.

IV AFTERCARE, REHABILITATION AND DAY CARE

ALLEN H (1981)
Voices of concern - a study of verbal communication about patients in a psychiatric day unit.
Journal of Advanced Nursing, vol 6, no 5, pp 355-362.

ARIE T (1979)
Day Care in Geriatric Psychiatry, 1978.
Age and Ageing, vol 8, no 4, pp 87-91.

ASHTON J R (1978)
Rehabilitation in psychiatry.
Community Health, vol 9, no 4, pp 216-220.
Through an examination of the literature, shows that the situation of rehabilitation for long-term patients is not a hopeless one, but that a commitment to rehabilitation involves more than slogans.

BAKER A A & BYRNE R J F (1977)
Another style of psychogeriatric service.
British Journal of Psychiatry, vol 130, pp 123-126.
Describes a psychogeriatric day hospital service in Gloucestershire where five per cent of admissions appear to have become long-stay.

234   Bibliography

BAKER G H B, WOODS T J & ANDERSON J A (1977)
Rehabilitation of the institutionalised patient.
British Journal of Psychiatry, vol 130, pp 484-488.

BENNETT D, FOX C, JOWELL T & SKINNER A C R (1976)
Towards a family approach in a psychiatric day hospital.
British Journal of Psychiatry, vol 129, pp 73-81.
Describes the effects of staff discussing their roles from the perspective of
family type dynamics; putting these ideas into practice for the treatment
programme within a day hospital.

BENNETT D H (1980)
District psychiatric rehabilitation.
World Hospitals, vol 16, no 4, pp 10-14.

BLUME R M, KAHN M & SACKS J (1979)
A collaborative day treatment programme for chronic patients in adult homes.
Hospital and Community Psychiatry, vol 30, no 1, pp 40-42.
Found that patients showed improved social behaviour as a result of training in
social and daily living skills, and that rates of rehospitalisation were
substantially reduced. However, clinical symptomatology remained unaltered.

BRANDON D (1980)
Cheap and cheerful: Knowsley Day Centre.
Mindout, no 43, pp 20-21.
Describes two low-cost day centres which could be copied elsewhere.

BRENNAN J O (1977)
The Welcome Club.
Nursing Times, vol 73, no II, p 393.
Describes a club introduced in order to help ex-patients make the transition
from hospital to the community

BURKE A W (1978)
Physical disorder among day hospital patients.
British Journal of Psychiatry, vol 133, pp 22-27.

CAMPBELL D (1976)
Community care of the mentally ill.
Focus, no 56, pp 13-14.
Provision of aftercare facilities by Scottish local authorities.

CAWLEY D & KELLY C (1978)
Day care complements hospitalisation.
Hospitals, vol 52, no 19, pp 141-142, 144.
A programme of day care for psychiatric patients can reduce costs and provide a
more suitable environment for treatment than inpatient care.

CASTLE STREET CIRCULAR (1978)
Day care launched.
Liverpool Council for Voluntary Service, no 103, pp 1-2.

COBB J (1980)
Tottenham Mews Day Hospital: a profile.
Nursing Focus, vol 1, no 8, pp 309-311.
Describes the varied work of a day hospital in an inner city area.

COLLICUTT J & JOYNER A (1980)
Adjusting to the new face of life.
Social Work Today, vol 11, no 48, pp 10-12.
Discusses the benefits that social skills training can offer psychiatric
patients with interpersonal difficulties who are going back into society.

DHSS (1978)
Report of a seminar on day care for the mentally ill.
King's Fund, mimeo.
Presents a number of papers about the development of day care with a particular
reference to the role of social services departments.

DHSS (1980)
Day care for the mentally ill - a discussion paper.
DHSS, mimeo.
An important review of policy and practices in day care for mentally ill
people.

ENTICKNAP B (1978)
Harlow House.
Nursing Times, vol 74, no 2, pp 1121-1124.
The work of Harlow House day hospital in Wycombe.

FAIRCLOUGH F (1978)
Community and day hospital care.
Nursing Mirror, vol 143, no 6, pp 67-68.
Discusses the value of the day hospital as an element of psychiatric care.

FOSTER A (1978)
In Practice.
Community Care, no 226, p 15.
Describes the creation of a club to help dependent patients achieve greater
independence despite their conviction that they are incapable of normal life.

FOTTRELL E, SPY T, MEARNS G, MACLEAN F & FOGARTY M (1980)
'Asset stripping' the declining mental hospital.
British Medical Journal, vol 280, pp 89-90.
Describes the development of a psychogeriatric day hospital from a long-stay
back-ward of a large mental hospital whose population of patients has decreased
by half.

GREEN J G & TIMBURY G C (1979)
A geriatric psychiatry day hospital service.
Age and Ageing, vol 8, no 1, pp 49-53.
Reviews the work of a day care unit for psychogeriatric patients. Finds that
the unit's main function has become that of providing an immediate, short-term
supportive facility for demented patients, mainly in the 75 and over age group,
and to their relatives, until such time as beds in long-stay psychogeriatric
wards become available.

GUIDRY L S, WINSTEAD D K, LEVINE M & EICKE F J (1979)
Evaluation of day treatment center effectiveness.
Journal of Clinical Psychiatry, vol 40, no 5, pp 221-224.
Prevention of hospitalisations and reduction of average length of stay when
admission unavoidable.

HARGREAVES R (1978)
Brindle House: an alternative structure for the mental health service.
Social Work Today, vol 9, no 43, pp 21-22.
Describes a community mental health service which integrates the skills of
various professions.

HARPER G (1980)
Driving force behind day care for the mentally ill.
Health and Social Service Journal, vol 90, pp 88-89.
Description of The Croft, Ripley, Derbyshire.

HASSANYEH F & DAVISON K (1981)
The psychiatric day hospital.
The Practitioner, vol 225, no 1362, pp 1825-1828.
Brief history of day hospitals which also describes the work of the day
hospital at Newcastle General Hospital.

HIGGINS P (1980)
A mobile day unit.
Nursing Times, vol 76, no 24, pp 1062-1064.

HOLLAND L K & WHALLEY M J (1981)
The work of the psychiatrist in a rehabilitation hospital.
British Journal of Psychiatry, vol 138, pp 222-229.
Describes the work a psychiatrist can do in helping staff to assist patients
who have been recently physically disabled and are suffering emotional
problems.

HOSPITAL DEVELOPMENT (1983)
Evesham Day Hospital.
Hospital Development, vol 11, no 1, p 13.
Describes the plan of the hospital which is one component in the overall
Worcester Development Plan.

HOWAT J G M & KOTNY E L (1982)
The outcome for discharged Nottingham long-stay in-patients.
British Journal of Psychiatry, vol 141, pp 590-594.
Follow-up of a large number of long-stay inpatients who were discharged showed
a high rate of readmissions but also much subsequent re-discharge and low
overall dependence on inpatient services. There was a high uptake of other
forms of support, especially day care, but little evidence of further movement
towards independence.

HUNTER E (1980)
Tilting at windmills.
New Society, vol 53, no 928, p 410.
A brief review of aftercare facilities for ex-patients in Scotland.

INGRAM J A (1978)
Who cares?
Royal Society of Health Journal, vol 98, no 3, pp 108-112.
Examines the non-availability of comprehensive rehabilitation services for
mental illness.

JONES I G & MUNBODH R (1982)
Evaluation of a day hospital for the demented elderly.
Health Bulletin, vol 40, no I, pp 10-15.

KELLY J A, PATTERSON J & SNOWDEN E (1979)
A pragmatic approach to mental health aftercare and partial hospitalisation.
Social Work in Health Care, vol 4, no 4, pp 431-443.

KILROY-SILK R (1979)
Now is the hour for action.
Health and Social Service Journal, vol LXXXIX, no 4656, p 1075.
Reviews lack of progress in day care facilities.

KNIGHT L & MURRAY J (1976)
Ready to leave? A survey of rehabilitation and aftercare for mentally ill
patients.
Community Care, no 116, pp 16-24.
Report of one of the most wide-ranging surveys ever conducted into rehabilitation and aftercare facilities. More than one third of NHS psychiatric
hospitals are covered.

LAKE B (1982)
An occupational therapist's view of day care for the elderly mentally ill.
British Journal of Occupational Therapy, vol 45, no 6, pp 205-208.

MEDICAL NEWS (1976)
Restaurant Club for mental patients helps rehabilitation.
Medical News, vol 8, no 12, p 16.

MARTIN S (1980)
No compromise - day care in its own right.
Social Work Today, vol 11, no 23, pp 13-14.
The work of Malvern Day Centre.

MIND (1981)
New   directions   for   psychiatric   day services: a report of a MIND conference
held   in   1980.
Presents   important   papers on the different uses of day care.

MITCHELL R G (1976)
Psychiatric day centres - a sound investment.
Nursing Times, vol 72, no 16, p 634.
Argues that day care has proved its effectiveness and decreases both the cost
of treatment and the stigma attached to mental illness.

MITCHELL S F & BIRLEY J L T (1983)
The use of ward support by psychiatric patients in the community.
British Journal of Psychiatry, vol 142, pp 9-15.
Describes a system of ward support for chronic psychiatric patients in an urban
community,   which makes available ward and staff facilities throughout the
24 hours and at weekends.

MUENCH H (1979)
Advantages of psychiatric day care.
Dimensions in Health Services, vol 56, no 2, pp 39-40.

MURRAY N (1981)
Working together in Warrington.
Community Care, no 392, p 9.
Account of the Warrington Day Centre Project supported by the local authority,
the Area Health Authority, MIND and the National Schizophrenia Fellowship. Has
a policy of open referral so that anyone suffering from psychiatric problems
can come in 'off the street'.

NORMAN B (1978)
An action team in Birmingham.
Social Work Service, no 15, pp 26-28.
Account of the work of an action team of social workers which is responsible
for supporting discharged psychiatric patients

NURSING TIMES (1981)
Psychiatric hospitals named as centres for rehabilitation.
Nursing Times, vol 77, no 43, p 1866.
Reports the government's designation of four psychiatric hospitals - Mapperley
Hospital,   Nottingham; Netherne Hospital, near Redhill, Surrey; St. Crispin's
Hospital, Northampton; Maudsley Hospital, Camberwell, London - as the first
demonstration centres for the rehabilitation of mentally ill patients.

PEACE S M (1982)
Review of day hospital provision in psychogeriatrics.
Health Trends, vol 14, no 4, pp 92-95.
Presents an overview of the current provision of day hospitals for the elderly
mentally ill.

PENK W E, CHARLES H L & VAN HOOSE T A (1978)
Comparative effectiveness of day hospital and inpatient psychiatric treatment.
Journal of Consulting and Clinical Psychology, vol 45, no 1, pp 94-101.
Findings which indicate that day care is an attractive alternative to inpatient
treatment.

PHILIP A E & MOORE J W (1976)
A job rating scale for use in rehabilitation.
British Journal of Psychiatry, vol 128, pp 462-466.
The development and use of a job rating scale which parallels the use of
patient assessment instruments.

PHILIP A E (1979)
Prediction of successful rehabilitation by nurse rating scale.
British Journal of Psychiatry, vol 134, pp 422-426.

PHILLIPS H (1982)
The challenge of setting up a day hospital for the elderly mentally ill.
British Journal of Occupational Therapy, vol 45, no 7, pp 239-241.

PLATT S D, KNIGHTS A C & HIRSCH S R (1980)
Caution and conservatism in the use of a psychiatric day hospital. Evidence
from a research project that failed.
Psychiatry Research, vol 3, no 2, pp 123-132.
The study sought to compare day care against inpatient care, but too few
patients in the acute phase of illness were referred to the day hospital. This
indicated that staff saw the two treatment settings as serving distinct but not
alternative functions.

PRECHNER M & PERRY B (1982)
The Heatherwood Day Centre.
British Journal of Occupational Therapy, vol 45, no 3, pp 81-82.

PRICE I G (1982)
An expanding 'Stage Army' of long-stay psychiatric patients.
British Journal of Psychiatry, vol 141, pp 595-601.
Analysis of contacts of patients with a large urban day hospital over a decade.

QUERY J M N (1980)
The rehabilitation hospital: a ten-year study of chronic psychiatric patients.
American Journal of Orthopsychiatry, vol 50, no 1, pp 156-159.
Study of the social functioning achieved by a cohort of chronically
hospitalised psychiatric patients who were placed in an intensive, total-push,
open hospital.

ROONEY P & MATHEWS R (1980)
Worcester Development Project for mentally ill people. Day Centres: policy and
user reaction.
Mental Health Building Evaluation Report No 2.
DHSS, London.

THE ROYAL COLLEGE OF PSYCHIATRISTS (1980)
Psychiatric Rehabilitation in the 1980's.
Report on rehabilitation from a working party of the social and community
psychiatry section. Considers facilities for rehabilitation of chronic
patients, including those resident in mental hospitals, and makes detailed
recommendations relating to the development of a comprehensive service.

SEELYE A (1980)
Day Centres for the mentally ill in adapted premises.
Medical Architecture Research Unit, Polytechnic of North London, for the DHSS.
Research project on the suitability of adapted premises for use as day centres.
Investigated 33 day centres sited in houses, churches, schools, shops, halls
and factories.

SEELYE A (1982)
The MARU study of day centres for the mentally ill in adapted premises.
Social Work Today, no 29, pp 5-7.
From the survey (see previous reference) concludes: "day centres can be
established with relatively minor modificatons, and day centres so created may
have features which can be regarded as positive advantages."

SHEAR M K & GILMORE N M (1979)
Case 4: the day hospital treatment of a schizophrenic patient.
Psychiatric Quarterly, vol 51, no 2, pp 161-166.

SHEPHERD G & RICHARDSON A (1979)
Organisation and interaction in psychiatric day centres.
Psychological Medicine, vol 9, no 3, pp 573-579.

SHIRES J (1977)
A travelling day hospital: an experiment in rural community psychiatric care.
Social Work Today, vol 28, no 24, pp 16-18.
Account of a novel scheme designed to provide service in rural areas, which
brings the clinical team to the patients' own small market town on a sessional
basis, and which the author believes to have a number of advantages over more
conventional provision.

SMITH C J (1978)
Recidivism and community adjustment amongst former mental patients.
Social Science and Medicine, vol 12, pp 17-27.

STEPHENS A & NATTRESS P (1978)
A study of day centres.
MIND, London.

THOMAS J (1980)
Psychiatrist who takes his clinic to the patient's doorstep.
Doctor, vol 10, no 24, p 36.
Describes Dr. Donald Dick's travelling psychiatric day hospital which services
a scattered rural area in Dorset.

TOKE E & CLEWS D (1977)
The function and effectiveness of a local authority day centre in the
rehabilitation of psychiatric conditions.
Occupational Therapy, vol 40, no 4, pp 75-78.
A detailed account of the anatomy and functions of a day centre.

TURNER-SMITH A & THOMSON I G (1979)
Patients' opinions: a survey of the effectiveness of a psychiatric day
hospital.
Nursing Times, vol 75, no 16, pp 675-679.

TYRER P J & REMINGTON M (1979)
Controlled comparison of day hospital and outpatient treatment for neurotic
disorders.
The Lancet, vol I, pp 1014-1016.
Showed no important differences in the outcome of day care and outpatient
treatment, although patients were more satisfied with the outpatient service.

WASHBURN S, VANNICELLI M, LONGBAUGH R & SCHEFF B-J (1976)
A controlled comparison of psychiatric day treatment and outpatient
hospitalisation.
Journal of Consulting and Clinical Psychology, vol 44, no 4, pp 665-675.
Shows that day patient treatment is, on the whole, superior to inpatient
treatment in five distinct areas: subjective distress, community functioning,
family burden, total hospital cost and days of attachment to the hospital
programme.

WATTS F N & BENNETT D H (1978)
Social deviance in a day hospital.
British Journal of Psychiatry, vol 132, pp 455-462.

WEIGHTMAN G (1977)
The road back to town.
New Society, vol 39, no 752, pp 440-441.
Describes an unusually thorough scheme in West Dorset which has succeeded in
helping patients back into the community.

WELDON E & FRANCES A (1977)
The day hospital: structures and functions.
Psychiatric Quarterly, vol 49, no 4, pp 338-342.
Authors suggest that a day hospital may serve as 1) an alternative to
hospitalisation or to shorten hospital stays, 2) as a long-term resocialization
experience, and 3) as an intense brief therapy environment.

WELDON E, CLARKIN J E, HENNESSY J J & FRANCES A (1979)
Day hospital versus outpatient treatment: a controlled study.
Psychiatric Quarterly, vol 51, no 2, pp 144-150.
Compares day hospital and outpatient treatment in relation to rehospitalisation, symptomatology, mood, community and vocational adjustment for 30
recently discharged patients with schizophrenic illness. Results show that day
hospital patients were significantly more involved in work and training
activities, but there were no significant differences in the other areas
measured.

WEYMAN A (1977)
Maximising care potential.
Health and Social Service Journal, vol LXXXVII, no 4542, p 829.
Describes the work of the Marlborough Day Hospital based in St. John's Wood and
founded in 1946.

WILDER J (1978)
An aid to community care.
Psychiatric Rehabilitation Association, London.
A teaching manual for those involved with the rehabilitation of psychiatric
patients in the community.

WILDER J (1982)
The day centre's role in psychiatric rehabilitation.
Therapy, vol 8, no 37, p 4.

WILSON D (1977)
Better day by day.
Pulse vol 34, no 14, p 16.
An account of the work of the Penge Psychiatric Day Unit.

V RESIDENTIAL CARE AND OCCUPATION

ABRAHAMSON D ET AL. (1979)
The good life at Goodmayes.
Health and Social Service Journal, vol LXXXIX, no 4643, pp 633-635.
Describes a rehabilitation project based at Goodmayes Hospital.

ANSTEE B H (1978)
An alternative to group homes.
British Journal of Psychiatry, vol 132, pp 356-360.
Describes a supported lodgings scheme as an alternative to traditional group
homes.

BROADHEAD E & WATSON M (1981)
A year in the life of an enclave.
Industrial Therapy, vol 6, no 2, pp 9-11.
Discusses the work of a working enclave - a group of severely disabled people
working under supervision in an ordinary and undifferentiated environment.

BUDSON R D (1978)
The psychiatric half-way house: a handbook of theory and practice.
University of Pittsburgh Press, Pittsburgh, USA.

CHICK J (1979)
Sheltered accommodation in the community mental health service in the 13th
arrondisement, Paris.
British Journal of Psychiatry, vol 135, pp 315-320.
Describes the use of sheltered accommodation in this part of Paris and suggests
that the need for such accommodation in the UK may be greater than the DHSS has
estimated.

CLARKE P (1979)
Accommodation - an aspect of community care for the mentally ill.
Scottish Association for Mental Health.

CORBALAN P & LUNING P (1979)
Fostering independence by groupwork in a residential setting.
Social Services, vol 8, no 11, pp 5,8.

CRESDEE D (1979)
Stepping-stones back to living at home.
CHC News, no 45, p 13.
Describes the work of Goodmayes Hospital in opening group homes for long-stay
patients in London Boroughs of Redbridge and Newham.

CRINE A (1981)
Portugal Prints - designs for the future.
Mindout, no 54, pp 20-21.
Reports on the rehabilitation workshop run by Westminster Association for
Mental Health.

CRINE A (1981)
Is the MSC abandoning the mentally disabled?
Mindout, no 53, pp 4-5.

CRINE A (1981)
Halfway house to independence.
Mindout, no 46, pp 10-13.
Report of a bed-sit scheme for young people run by Tyneside Association for
Mental Health.

CRINE A (1981)
Disabled and unemployed.
Mindout, no 46.
Argues that employment opportunities for the mentally disabled range from
patchy to non-existent.

DORSET AHA (1977)
The Kings Park Hospital at Home: an option for the East Dorset Health Care
District. mimeo.
Considers the possibility of introducing the 'Hospital at Home' concept as
developed in France for the care of the elderly mentally ill. The aim of this
type of service is to allow patients to remain at home, yet at the same time
receive care equal to that of a traditional hospital. The scheme avoids the
expenditure involved in building and maintaining traditional hospitals.

DURRANT B W (1976)
Back to the community with a hospital-made family.
Health and Social Service Journal, vol LXXXVI, no 4506, pp 1592-1593.
Account of a scheme at Oakwood Hospital, Maidstone, for the training and
placement of psychiatric patients as family groups in private homes in the
community.

ETHERINGTON S (1983)
Housing and Mental Health.
MIND in association with Circle 33 Housing Trust.

FLETCHER P (1980)
Work for minds on the mend.
Health and Social Service Journal, vol LXXXX, no 4701, pp 909-910.
Describes 'Restore', a pioneer scheme in Oxford, which provides a new approach
to the provision of sheltered work for the mentally disabled.

FRANEY R (1979)
Public virtues, private vices.
Roof, vol 4, no 6, pp 178-181.
Report of hostels for the mentally disordered in Birmingham.

GARIOCH G (1978)
Mental health hostels - a waste of money?
Social Work Today, vol 9, no 42, p 26.
Questions the value of building mini-institutions when clients could be placed
in hotels and guest houses or live in group homes, involving no capital outlay,
and far less in terms of running costs.

GODBER C (1978)
Kinloss Court: an experiment in sheltered housing and collaboration.
Social Work Service, no 45, pp 42-45.

GOLDSTONE L A & TOOLEY D M (1976)
Aspects of hostel facilities for the mentally ill in Greater Manchester.
Community Health, vol 8, no 2, pp 86-94.

GREEN L (1980)
The factory with a difference.
BMA News Review, vol 6, no 10, pp 80-85.
Describes the work of the Industrial Therapy Organisation (Thames) Ltd in West
London where the workers are all ex-patients or have psychiatric problems.

HEGINBOTHAM C (1982)
Housing management, social work and mental illness.
King's Fund Centre, London.
Conference papers dealing with both preventive and rehabilitative aspects of
housing provision with an emphasis on co-ordination between health, social
services and housing agencies.

HENDRY M (1981)
Charting the return to work.
Therapy, vol 8, no 20, p 3.
Report of a scheme at Severalls Hospital, Essex, designed to gear patients for
the working environment.

HENNIGAN M & DEMARESQ D (1978)
The Camden adult care scheme.
Social Work Service, no 15, pp 19-22.

HUGHES D (1978)
How psychiatric patients manage out of hospital. Community provision, living
standards and financial needs.
The Disability Alliance in conjunction with the Mental Health Foundation.

LEADER M A (1978)
The Hillside aftercare apartment project: a pilot follow-up study.
Social Work in Health Care, vol 3, no 4, pp 419-429.
Evaluation of a project.

LEOPOLDT H & McSTAY P (1980)
The psychiatric group home - 2.
Nursing Times, vol 76, no 20, pp 866-868.
Outline of the support and management system of the Oxford Group Home
organisation.

KLEIN R (1979)
Making your own home.
Mindout, no 34, p 24.
Describes a bedsitter scheme for ex-patients in Croydon undertaken by MIND.

KNIGHT L (1981)
Aspects of rehabilitation: Fountain House.
Mindout, no 47, pp 17-19.
A club in New York for ex-mental patients which offers exciting example for
other countries.

KNIGHT L (1977)
Working back to dignity.
Community Care, no 183, pp 20-22.
Describes the work at Netherne Hospital in Surrey, which has earned a high
reputation for its rehabilitative methods. Also highlights the lack of
facilities in the community.

MARTIN D (1979)
Family care for the mentally disordered in Belgium.
Health and Social Service Journal, vol LXXXIX, no 4671, pp C33-C40.
Report of a project whose aim was to discover the strengths and weaknesses of
family care - fostering - for mentally, physically, socially or emotionally
handicapped adults. Suitable clients might be in hospital or residental care,
or gravely at risk in the community. Emphasis on the use of ordinary families
as social service resources.

MAYERS G (1980)
A refuge in West London.
Voluntary Housing, vol 12, no 3, p 7.

McANDREW C H, OVERTON N K & WHYTE M (1980)
Life in the community: a survey of the Prestwich Hospital group homes,
Psychiatric Rehabilitation Association, London.

McDONALD C (1979)
How we rehabilitated 42 long-stay psychiatric patients.
Geriatric Medicine, vol 9, no 6, pp 53-54,57.
A rehabilitation programme for 'graduate' patients who had grown old in a
psychiatric hospital resulted in 42 discharges into residential places. The
scheme involved the officers of the homes attending ward rounds during the
assessment period and continuing follow-up by psychogeriatric nurses.

MEACHER M (1976)
After one and half million years in hospital.....
Social Work Today, vol 7, no 6, p 1623.
Outlines a range of residential services which are provided and could be
provided despite the economic recession.

MIND REPORT (1976)
The next step: community care for former psychiatric patients in six towns.
Profiles of services in Bristol, Gateshead, Newcastle-upon-Tyne, Sheffield,
Oldham and Portsmouth.

MIND (1976)
You can't have one without the other.
Report on the integration of a hospital-based rehabilitation scheme and a
community-based resettlement project in North Gwent.

MIND (1977)
Home from hospital: progress and results.
Report of the progress of the MIND campaign aimed at increasing the amount of
caring accommodation in the community for former psychiatric patients.

MIND REPORT (1977)
A new home in a New Town.
A survey of how 20 New Town Development Corporations are tackling the task of
housing people discharged from psychiatric hospitals.

MIND REPORT 15 (1978)
Room to let: report on nine social service lodgings schemes.
Schemes included are: The Old Manor Hospital, Salisbury, Croydon SSD,
Wandsworth SSD, North Yorkshire SSD, Lambeth SSD, Herrison Hospital, Dorset,
Manchester SSD, Kent SSD, Camden SSD. Also includes a list of schemes in
England and Wales.

MIND (1979)
Allies on the touchline.
Report on the potential for co-operation between Housing Associations, the
responsible statutory authorities and voluntary organisations in the task of
re-housing ex-psychiatric patients.

MIND (1979)
Off the waiting list.
Report on the forging of links between District Housing Authorities in Dyfed
and the rehabilitation team at St. David's Hospital, Carmarthen, leading to the
resettlement in the community of long-term psychiatric patients.

MINDOUT (1978)
One step up.....and two steps down.
Mindout, no 29, pp 12-15.
An excellent guide for psychiatric patients going back to work.

NATIONAL ASSOCIATION OF VOLUNTARY HOSTELS & MIND (1980)
Handbook of access to special housing for mentally ill and mentally
handicapped adults in Greater London.
NAVH & MIND.

NURSING TIMES (1976)
Brent finds an answer.
Nursing Times, vol 72, no 44, p 1700.
Self-contained flatlets with a housing association tenancy.

OLSEN M R (1979)
The care of the mentally disordered: an examination of some alternatives to
hospital care.
BASW, London.
The contributors examine the evidence for and against aftercare for chronic
psychiatric patients in non-hospital environments. They also describe the
outcome of investigations and research into alternatives including care in day
centres, hostels, group homes, boarding houses, and substitute family care.
Finally, they examine the role of local authorities and the voluntary sector in
such schemes.

PARK F et al. (1980)
Meeting the needs of the mentally ill: one solution.
Voluntary Housing, vol 12, no 9, pp 15-17.
A housing scheme for psychiatric patients in Kensington.

PRAGER C (1979)
A refuge in West London.
Mindout, no 33, p 24.
Account of a half-way house set up by Kensington and Chelsea MIND.

PRITLOVE J H (1976)
Evaluating a group home: problems and results.
British Journal of Social Work, vol 6, no 3, pp 353-376.
Discusses the need for an evaluative framework for group homes for the mentally
ill.

PRITLOVE J H (1976)
We don't harm one another: an evaluation of the first three years of a group
home for ex-psychiatric patients in a northern city.
The author, Keighley.

PRITLOVE J H (1983)
Accommodation without resident staff for ex-psychiatric patients: changing
trends and needs.
British Journal of Social Work, vol 13, no 1, pp 75-92.
Describes a survey of such accommodation in a Metropolitan local authority area
carried out in 1977-78 which shows that population is beginning to include both
elderly, institutionalised and chronically handicapped group and a younger,
more lively group.

PRYCE I G (1977)
The selection of long-stay hospital patients for hostels: a study of patients
selected for an experimental hostel and for local authority hostels.
Psychological Medicine, vol 7, no 2, pp 331-343.

PURCELL R (1980)
Housing and mental health.
Design for Special Needs, no 23, p 2.
Report of a conference on housing management, social work and mental illness.

RICHIE J, KEEGAN J, & BOSANQUET N (1983)
Housing for mentally ill and mentally handicapped people.
DoE, HMSO.
Research study which is a profile of the amount and type of accommodation
provided by local housing authorities, housing associations and voluntary
organisations. Also contains case studies which review and assess different
forms of provision with respect to development, organisation and support.
Financial profile included.

ROSS G (1981)
Lifestyle of long-term psychiatric patients in the London Borough of Hackney.
Psychiatric Rehabilitation Association.
Survey of 100 patients with chronic psychiatric illness.

THE ROYAL BOROUGH OF KENSINGTON AND CHELSEA (1979)
Research report: Accommodation needs of the mentally ill.
Social Services Department.

RYAN P & HEWETT S (1976)
A pilot study of hostels for the mentally ill.
Social Work Today, vol 6, no 25, pp 774-778.
Based on a study of 76 residents of non-hospital accommodation. Suggests that
there is a need for a new kind of hostel, geared specifically to the needs of
the new long-term population.

SCHOFIELD J & PATTERSON D (1979)
Group homes: a recipe for community living.
British Journal of Occupational Therapy, vol 42, no 11, pp 278-279.

SEELYE A (1976)
Hostels for the mentally ill in ordinary houses.
The Medical Architecture Unit, Polytechnic of North London, for the DHSS.
Describes a project set up to appraise the suitability and adaptability of
different generic housing types for hostel purposes.

SEELYE A (1978)
The use of ordinary housing for hostels for the mentally ill.
Social Work Service, no 15, pp 45-48.

SEGAL S P (1979)
Sheltered care needs of the mentally ill.
Health and Social Work, vol 4, pp 41-57.

SNAP (1976)
Putting rehabilitation into practice.
SNAP, September, p 29.
Describes the work originating at Middlewood Hospital in rehabilitating
long-stay patients.

STEVENS P (1982)
Herrison - a social worker's point of view.
Growth Point, no 11, pp 4-5.
Describes the work taking place at the Herrison Hospital Therapeutic Farm in
Dorset.

TARLO H (1981)
Don't take their initiative away.
Community Care, no 367, pp 18-20.
Two therapeutic communities at Droitwich.

TATTERSALL W (1978)
Housing allocation help.
Social Work Service, no 15, p 38-40.
Presents the role of Housing Associations in providing accommodation for
psychiatric patients.

THORNICROFT G (1979)
Group homes: is the enthusiasm justified?
Pulse, vol 39, no 1, pp 34-35.
Argues that the current range of rehabilitative facilities should be expanded
if community care is to bear any credibility.

TUCKER D (1980)
A special housing project for ex-psychiatric patients.
Housing Review, vol 29, no 2, pp 43-44.
Report of a project in Kensington.

WALKER L G (1979)
The effect of some incentives on the work performance of psychiatric patients
at a rehabilitation workshop.
British Journal of Psychiatry, vol 134, pp 427-435.

WANSBOROUGH N & COOPER P (1980)
Open employment after mental illness.
Tavistock, London.

SUBJECT INDEX

accessibility
 information 32-4
 services 83
accommodation 84,130
 communal 94
 interim secure 122
 Part III 194
 semi-secure 79
 size of schemes 103
 with support 94, 108,
  109, 127, 205, 208
accountability 116, 207
achievements 130
administrator 59, 164-70
admission
 change of status 68
 reductions 87
alcohol
 problems 142
 services 130
anti-psychiatrists 57-8,
 62
anxiety 59, 69, 180
assessment 172, 205
 joint 158
 use of service 105
asylum 48, 77-8, 87
attachment schemes in
 general practice 183
attitudes 16, 27, 78, 82,
 92, 97, 99, 117, 132

Barclay Report 208
beds 21, 80, 85, 106-9

behaviour 59, 63, 68
beneficence 44-9
Bethlem Hospital 123
Better Services for the
 Mentally Ill 21, 79,
 106, 154, 171
Birmingham 154, 162
Birmingham Association
 for Mental Health 158,
 162
Black Report 201
Bloomsbury 118
Brindle House 81, 171
Broadmoor Hospital 121
budget, budgeting 112,
 205, 207
Butler Committee 121

Camden 106
capital 146
Care in the Community in-
 itiative (see also
 joint finance) 22,
 25-6, 83, 167, 206
care, long-term 83, 191
change
 impetus 14
 pace 151
 preconditions 132
Charles Davis House 162
Cinderella 13-5, 72, 164,
 211
City and Hackney 14, 79,
 87, 106, 111, 128, 164

City and Hackney Assoc-
    iation for Mental
    Health 95, 130
Claybury Hospital 86
closure of hospitals 22,
    86, 207
cluster flats 95
collaboration 15, 23,
    102, 132-3, 148,
    150-1, 160, 194, 208,
    212
communication 23, 130,
    158, 166
community care 35, 55,
    79, 84, 124, 143, 153,
    209
    cost 208
Community Health Council
    86, 92, 108
community psychiatric
    nurses, nursing serv-
    ice 22-3, 84, 99, 107,
    114, 130, 175
community psychiatry
    39, 47, 55
    posts 41
Community Psychiatry Res-
    earch Unit (CPRU) 13,
    24, 92, 95, 98, 129,
    146
confidentiality 51
contract, carer and
    client 49
co-operation
    obstacles 156-7
    practical aspects
    157-9
co-ordination 15, 129,
    130, 135, 144
Copec Housing Trust 162
costing systems 111
costs 36
    and benefits 47-8
counselling 174, 181
crisis intervention 81,
    173
cycle of development 144

day care 109, 162, 177,
    193
day centre 154, 176, 208

day hospital 21, 81, 106,
    191-6
definitions of housing
    schemes 103
dementia 191-6
Department of the Envir-
    onment 14, 101, 167,
    207
depression 180
DGH units 21-3, 61, 65,
    68, 86-7
diagnosis 50
    training in 40
difficulties (see also
    problems) 162, 212
disability 39, 91, 128,
    175
    gap 131, 134
district general hospital
    (see DGH units)
duty 52

ECT 37, 50
education 54, 151, 154,
    165, 170, 201-2
elderly 24, 191-6
emergencies, emergency
    service 42, 52, 81,
    130, 174, 176, 209
ethics 44-54
evaluation 147, 159, 176
    of hostels 25
experiment 25, 28

families 41-2, 54, 71,
    160, 212
finance (see also joint
    finance, funding,
    money) 16, 92
flatshare scheme 84, 95
flexibility 95-6, 134,
    149
    of funding 99, 132
Flint Green House 162
forecasting 31, 108
Friern Hospital 86
funding 99, 117, 132-3,
    166-8, 206-7

gap 84, 104, 129, 145,
    208

gap
    disability 131, 134
Gatsby Trust 13, 84, 129,
    133
general hospitals (see
    DGH units)
general practice (see
    also GPs) 25, 35,
    118, 175, 178-87
    and social workers
    182-4
    attachment schemes 183
Glancy Report 122,125
Glossop 171
goals 60,64
Goodmayes Hospital 105
Good Practices in Mental
    Health Project (GPMH)
    26, 89, 132, 145, 149
GPs (see also general
    practice) 107
    relationship with
    psychiatrists 185-7
group home 84, 95, 108

Hackney 84, 91, 123
Handen Road 81
Haringey 106
Health Advisory Service
    86
Health Education Council
    202
hierarchy 28, 82, 135,
    176
Highcroft Hospital 154,
    163
Hollymoor Hospital 154-63
Homerton Hospital 130
hospital
    closure 22, 86, 207
    nucleus 105
    zone 87
    mental (see mental
    hospital)
hostel 25, 84, 88, 94,
    154, 175
housing association 97,
    100-4
Housing Association Grant
    100
Housing Corporation 101

housing
    local authority 91
    managers 98
    medical assessments
    91
Hyde 171

information 91-2, 151,
    205
    accessibility 32-4
    computerised 37
    gaps 35-7, 123, 193,
    196
    linking 33, 37
    medication 163
    patients and services
    35-7
    policies 36-7, 51
    regional 32
    sources 34
    systems 29, 31, 145
Inner Cities Partnership
    99, 167
inner city 79, 126, 131
innovation 25, 29, 61,
    64, 84, 97, 104, 150
institutions
    as resource 146
    total 59
intensive care (see
    also Psychiatric int-
    ensive care unit)
    122-7
interfaces 129, 132, 135
interviews 70, 107
Islington 106
Italy 64

joint
    assessment 158
    finance (see also
    Care in the Community)
    25, 112, 153, 166-7
    funding 99, 101, 99
    planning 23, 92, 113,
    144, 146, 169-70, 204
    system 153, 173
justice 44-8

key
    therapist 173

key worker 116
Korner Report 36

label, labelled 68, 123,
    131, 150, 166
language 140, 158, 165,
    170
legal framework 201
lobbying 113, 168
London and Quadrant
    Housing Trust 95, 101
Long Grove Hospital 128

management
    committees 97, 101
    nursing 115
    service 144, 173, 204
Maudsley Hospital 88
medical sociology,
    sociologists 55, 67
Medidos system 163
mental hospital 22, 59,
    61-2, 65, 86, 118, 206
Mental Health Act
    1959 79, 121
    1983 201
Mental Health Enquiry
    (MHE) 31-2, 34-5
Mental Health Foundation
    129
mental health interest
    groups (see planning
    groups
mental illness hospital
    (see mental hospital)
Mental Illness Policy
    Paper 14
Mental Treatment Act 1939
    78
Middlewood House 154-63
MIND 14, 86, 150, 201
money 29, 95, 102, 146,
    148, 206
    labelling of 113
morbidity 34, 181
multidisciplinary team
    23, 28, 53, 94, 126,
    135, 159, 179

National Schizophrenia
    Fellowship 52, 160

need, needs
    accommodation 84
    assessment 92
    Bradshaw's taxonomy
    105
    expressed 105, 110
    intensive care 124
    occupation 84
    unexpressed 110
neurotic disorder 70
'new' long-stay (see
    patients)
Newham 105, 123
Newham Association for
    Mental Health 107
Nodder Report 22
non-discrimination (see
    also justice) 45
normalisation 200
normality 57, 63
norms 23, 80-1, 106, 145,
    205
nucleus hospital 105

obstacles to co-operation
    156-7
occupation 84-5, 109
occupational therapy 81
offenders 121, 124
Office of Population Cen-
    suses and Surveys 35
'old' long-stay (see
    patients)
Old People's Homes 193
Opportunities for Volun-
    teering 26

patients
    chronic 48, 82-5, 128
    flows 33, 207
    'new' long-stay 24-5,
    84-5, 88, 109, 136
    numbers 33
    'old' long-stay 82-5,
    107, 109
    rights 52, 200
    severely disturbed 123
    surveys 70, 83, 92,
    193
philosophy 93, 119,
    CPN service 117

PICU (Psychiatric Inten-
    sive Care Unit) 122-6
planning
    groups, teams 92, 113,
    129, 144-5
    operational 172
    processes 129, 144,
    146
    shopping list approach
    144, 168
    system 112, 203-4
policy
    about information 51
    DHSS 22
    housing association
    103
    joint system 161
    local 109
    'open door' 173
    regional 122, 125
Policy for Action 21
prevalence rates 178
prevention 202
primary care, health care
    (see general
    practice)
principles 28, 44-5, 52,
    133, 154, 172, 199
    and practice 27
priorities 108, 110, 133,
    146
    clashes of 98
    local 113
privacy 51
problems (see also
    difficulties, obst-
    acles) 175-6, 203
psychiatric hospital
    (see mental
    hospital)
Psychiatric Intensive
    Care Unit (PICU) 122-6
Psychiatric Rehabilit-
    ation Association
    (PRA) 132
psychiatric service
    register 14, 37
psychiatric unit (see
    DGH unit)
psychologist
    role 157

psychosocial
    counselling 174
    problems 181, 183
psychotropic drugs 179

readmission 128
    rates 85, 107
reciprocity 45
Redbridge 105
referral
    rate 176
    self- 173
    to specialist services
    185
rehabilitation 73, 81
    prisoners of war 78
    unit 154
    ward 158
rehousing 96
rejection 70-3
research 62-3, 69, 87,
    94, 127, 130, 134
    grants 168
    health service 29
responsibility 116
revenue 146
right, rights
    access 50
    individuals 49
    patients 52, 200
    to treatment 51
role, roles
    carer 53
    definitions 57
    ex-patient 69
    psychiatrist 184
    psychologist 157
    sick 62
    social 60
    staff 147
respect for persons 44
Runwell Hospital 86

schizophrenia 88, 96
security, secure
    facilities 24, 125
Seebohm Report 182
self-help groups 52, 89
self-referral 173

service, services
   accessibility 83
   assessment of use 105
   community 164
   dynamic aspects 32
   network 140
   non-acute 164
   planning 144
   transfer of 211
sheltered workshop, emp-
   loyment 175, 208
social
   control 53-9, 61-4
   factors 128, 179
   network 84, 131
   roles 60
   skills 85, 131
   worker
      recommendations 51
      and general prac-
      tice 182-4
Solihull 154
Southampton 70
special
   hospitals 79, 121
   projects 102, 134
specialty costing 111
staff 143, 161, 173, 192
staffing
   levels 117, 123
   rates 126
statistics 21-2, 31, 129
stigma, stigmatisation
   53, 63, 67, 96
strategy 141, 144-6, 156,
   166, 168
stress 202
superintendent 59, 89
support 94, 96, 98, 119
   community 83, 142, 195
   mobile team 99
   Network 13, 95, 130
   social 95

Tameside 171
timescale 167, 176, 207
Tooting Bec Hospital 123
top-slicing 113, 205
Tower Hamlets 106, 123
trainee 41-2

training 87, 126
   facilities 155
   nurses 115
   programmes 159
   techniques 156
transfer
   patients 207
   services 211
tribunals 26

Urban Aid (see Inner
   Cities Partnership)

values 44
Vanguard Commune 95, 102,
   130, 133
voluntary organisation
   (also agency, group,
   sector) 23, 92, 98,
   160, 175, 207
volunteers 26, 84, 89,
   149, 170, 209

wards 94, 123, 161, 171
   acute 88
   admission 88
   back 60
   long-stay 88, 118, 155
   191, 207
   psychogeriatric 191
   rehabilitation 158
Worcester project 25
World Health Organisation
   148

zone hospital 87